Helping Others with Depression

A JOHNS HOPKINS PRESS HEALTH BOOK

Helping Others with

DEPRESSION

WORDS TO SAY, THINGS TO DO

Susan J. Noonan, MD, MPH

Foreword by Maurizio Fava, MD,
and Timothy J. Petersen, PhD

JOHNS HOPKINS UNIVERSITY PRESS

Baltimore

Note to the Reader: This book is not meant to substitute for medical care of people who have depression or other mental disorders, and treatment should not be based solely on its contents. Instead, treatment must be developed in a dialogue between the individual and his or her physician. This book has been written to help with that dialogue.

If you or someone you know is thinking about suicide, immediately contact your health care provider, go to the nearest Emergency Department, or call 9-1-1.

Johns Hopkins University Press
2715 North Charles Street
Baltimore, Maryland 21218-4363
www.press.jhu.edu

Library of Congress Cataloging-in-Publication Data

Names: Noonan, Susan J., 1953– author.
Title: Helping others with depression : words to say, things to do / Susan J. Noonan,
    MD, MPH.
Description: Baltimore : Johns Hopkins University Press, [2020] | Series: A Johns Hopkins
    Press health book | Includes bibliographical references and index.
Identifiers: LCCN 2020005972 | ISBN 9781421439297 (hardcover) | ISBN 9781421439303
    (paperback) | ISBN 9781421439310 (ebook)
Subjects: LCSH: Depression, Mental. | Depression, Mental—Treatment.
Classification: LCC RC537 .N658 2021 | DDC 616.85/27—dc23
LC record available at https://lccn.loc.gov/2020005972

A catalog record for this book is available from the British Library.

Special discounts are available for bulk purchases of this book. For more information, please contact Special Sales at specialsales@press.jhu.edu.

Johns Hopkins University Press uses environmentally friendly book materials, including recycled text paper that is composed of at least 30 percent post-consumer waste, whenever possible.

Contents

Tables

Foreword

At any given time, over 250 million individuals worldwide suffer from depression. Although everyone experiences emotional distress resulting from such typical life stressors as traffic delays, interpersonal conflict, and work deadlines, these stressors are, for the most part, temporary. Depression is different than simple emotional distress in notable ways. It is characterized by significant symptoms that interfere with one's ability to function effectively in various areas of your life. Common symptoms of depression include depressed or "low" mood, decreased interest in normal activities, inability to experience pleasure, sleep and appetite disturbances, difficulty concentrating, low energy levels, and feelings of hopeless and helplessness.

Many times, individuals experience thoughts of suicide; annually, over 750,000 individuals worldwide die from suicide. In the United States, during the 10-year period from 2007 to 2017, rates of suicide in individuals aged 10 to 24 increased by 56%. In fact, in the United States, suicide has become the second leading cause of death for those between the ages of 10 and 34. Depression is an illness that also can affect physical health negatively. Having a heart condition, for example can increase your risk for depression and lead to worse outcomes if you are depressed.

Although there is an abundance of evidence-based treatments for depression, experts in the field of mental health are just beginning to understand what treatments work best for any given individual. Such personalized, customized treatment is one critical area of continued study, especially given the fact that only 30% to 40% of individuals respond favorably to an initial treatment for depression, whether it is in the form of medication, talk therapy, mind-body treatments, such as deep breathing exercises. Even with all of the various treatments available, the reality for most people with depression is that they will need more than one form of treatment before reaching remission. Research indicates that your likelihood of achieving remission lowers with each successive treatment trial, underscoring the need to better tailor treatments when first seeking treatment.

An additional challenge facing mental healthcare specialists is how to increase dissemination of evidence-based practices to practitioners and patients who may have limited access to this information. Given the growing reliance on virtual forms of knowledge transmission and misinformation widely available, it is more important than ever to ensure we are providing sound information related to the prevention, diagnosis, and treatment of depression. Practitioners and patients living and working in more remote areas will increasingly rely on information provided via podcasts, e-books, and e-journals.

Dr. Noonan's latest book, *Helping Others with Depression: Words to Say, Things to Do*, is a wonderful resource that is comprehensive and evidence-based. It provides practical information for individuals experiencing depression along with members of their social network, including family and friends, as well as to those on the front lines providing treatment for depression. Dr. Noonan, as both a physician and individual who has struggled with depression for many years, brings a unique voice and set of experiences to this book. Chapters are organized into broad themes including the assessment and accurate diagnosis of depression, navigation of the mental health care system, utilization of cognitive and behavioral strategies, understanding depression across age ranges, consideration of ways in which caregivers can be most effective, and the role of technology in mental health treatment. Dr. Noonan's writing style is highly accessible and the content is conveyed in a straightforward manner. Case examples are used effectively to illustrate important ideas and principles.

From our perspective as a practicing psychiatrist as well as a psychologist, we believe that this book is an important addition to the literature. Far too often, friends and family members of those who are experiencing depression report not knowing what to say or do to help. This book provides concrete details about how you can help, including finding the best way to communicate, when to intervene, and how you can be of assistance. We commend Dr. Noonan for continuing her efforts to provide helpful resources to all those who may be affected by depression.

Maurizio Fava, MD
Psychiatrist in Chief
Massachusetts General Hospital
Boston, MA

Timothy J. Petersen, PhD
Staff Psychologist
Massachusetts General Hospital
Boston, MA

Acknowledgments

It is with great fortune that I present to you my fourth book on managing depression. This would not be possible without the support of you, the readers, and those in my life who keep me afloat. I continue to owe my deepest thanks and gratitude to Drs. Andrew Nierenberg, Jonathan Alpert, Timothy Petersen, and Karen Carlson. My family has been generous and supportive, and for that I am most grateful. And my friends, the ones who have sustained me throughout, deserve immeasurable thanks and appreciation.

In addition, the insightful staff at Johns Hopkins University Press warrants particular recognition, including, but not limited to, my editors Joe Rusko, Juliana McCarthy, and Andre Barnett. They again guided me along this amazing journey with perceptive, meticulous, and thoughtful care. No book is published alone.

Helping Others with Depression

Introduction

If you've chosen to open this book, you're in the company of many like you who are searching for ways to help a family member or a close friend who has depression or bipolar disorder. It's designed for you. It will give you some ideas on what to say and do. It's also a companion volume to my book written for those who themselves are suffering with a mood disorder: *Take Control of Your Depression: Strategies to Help You Feel Better Now* (2018).

Perhaps in the past you've felt awkward trying to help someone with such an emotionally charged problem. Maybe you weren't sure how to respond. Some people feel uncomfortable bringing up sensitive issues and can be at a loss for words in these situations. It's normal to worry about saying or doing the "wrong" thing and perhaps making the situation worse. This is a common fear.

Perhaps you've tried to talk to your friend or family member who is depressed and have felt shut out or excluded. Perhaps you're afraid that whatever you do isn't going to be helpful or make a difference, even though you have good intentions. You are left feeling frustrated, powerless, and, eventually, worn out.

You may have found that some circumstances require a delicate touch—something with which you may not have had a lot of experience. In addition, if your family member is in a "hot zone" of emotion, he or she may not be thinking clearly. He may misinterpret what you say or do. This can happen in the best of relationships. This book will help guide you through those situations that require a heightened sensitivity or awareness of your loved one's distorted thinking.

If you're the parent of a teen or young adult who has a mood disorder, you may feel an added responsibility to guide and support him through this illness. You might discover that he does not want to share his struggles or is reluctant to seek treatment and wonder why. That's pretty common. You're put in a difficult position, and you may feel helpless, unable to do anything for your child. With an elderly parent who has depression, stubborn or old-school ways of regarding mental illness can interfere with effective care. When the problem is a mental illness, the stakes can be high.

My goal in writing this book is to bring depression-management strategies to those struggling to deal with this disabling illness in their spouse, sibling, parent, teenage or adult child, or close friend. I draw on personal experience as a patient, provider, and caretaker; on educational resources, including evidence-based research; on psychoeducational programs and seminars; on experts in the field; and on others' personal patient and family experiences. I offer recommendations on what to say and do when your family member or friend has depression-related difficulties. I also offer ways for you to foster resilience in those who have depression. Then I focus on you, the caregiver or supporter, who personally feels the stress of the illness. You need assistance during these times and must learn to care for yourself as well.

So what exactly are we talking about? Major depression and bipolar disorder are common biologically based conditions of the mind and body that affect the thoughts, feelings, actions, and everyday lives of many people. These two conditions are *mood disorders*, which by nature often are relapsing and remitting. This means that the symptoms can come and go over time in a pattern unique to each person. The fluctuations in your spouse's, child's, or parent's illness may make it tough to predict what each day will be like. These mood changes can be frustrating to observe and live with, and it may be hard to know how to handle them.

Mood disorders are considered among the most disabling of all medical conditions and are a huge burden across the globe; specifically, depression is the fourth leading "burden of disease or injury cause" worldwide and is a root cause of suicide and heart (cardiovascular) disease. Depression and bipolar disorder have an impact on nearly every level of an affected person's functioning, which in turn influences his or her quality of life. The degree of psychological and social disability they create is related to the severity of one's depression symptoms. In all cultures and societies, depression is associated with cognitive (thought) impairment, decreased function and productivity in daily life, and underperformance and higher absenteeism (missed days) in work and school. This may lead to decreased income or unemployment, fewer life opportunities, days lost because of illness, a lower quality of life, and a greater burden (both social and economic) to families and societies throughout the world. In addition, mood disorders can be disruptive to the stability of the family and may lead to separation or divorce. Depression in a parent has an effect on children in the family and has been linked with fetal and neonatal risks (such as premature births) and risks to normal child development through impaired parent-child bonding or attachment.

Depression affects about 300 million people of all ages worldwide (World Health Organization 2018). An estimated 16.2 million adults and 3.1 million adolescents aged 12 to 17 experienced at least one major depressive episode in the United States in 2016 (National Institute of Mental Health [NIMH] 2018). Trends show that these numbers are increasing. In addition, approximately one-third of adults and almost two-thirds of adolescents who experience depression do not receive any professional mental health treatment (NIMH 2016). Bipolar disorder (bipolar I, II, and bipolar spectrum) affects another 4.5 percent of adults at some time in their lives and 2.9 percent of adolescents.

These large numbers may be surprising to you. People often hide their illness and do not speak openly of it for a variety of reasons. The fear of stigmatization—being unfairly labeled or stereotyped—is the most common. Stigma, or unfounded judgment and criticism based on misinformation, upsets the lives of many people who have mental illness and causes great distress. Even though great strides have been made in understanding mood disorders as a medical condition, those affected still face social and workplace discrimination.

While sitting in a roundtable discussion on mood disorders with parents, spouses, and patients at Massachusetts General Hospital in Boston, I heard the frustration of supporters of those who have depression and bipolar disorder. Family members and close friends are usually the first to recognize the symptoms of depression and the ones providing daily support. Most felt powerless to know what steps to take, what to say or do in response to symptoms, or how to change the course of the illness. I saw them struggle, too, with the unpredictable nature of mood disorders. I know firsthand that many family members and friends are looking for information on how to respond to the ups and downs of a loved one's mood disorder but have few places to go for guidance on how to help.

This book is full of ideas for you to try. Some may work for you and your friend or family member; some may not. Not all families and relationships are alike or interact in the same way. You have to do what feels right for both of you. While there are similarities in how people experience depression, everyone is different. Each person also has their own way of communicating distress and accepting help. Some people are more private, some more talkative, and some more active. Attempt to understand your family member's unique style, reactions, and openness to receiving your help, and base your approach on that.

Try something from this book that you think may be helpful and see how he or she responds. Be careful not to force any one idea, especially if it causes more agitation or withdrawal. If you find that one approach doesn't work, use another. Or change it slightly and try it on another day. For example, if your spouse gets angry when you bring up his depression or if he considers it intrusive when you ask about his problems or how he is feeling, then stop and try a different approach. If he doesn't want to talk today, perhaps he'll go for a bike ride or a long walk with you. He may be ready to talk another day. Remember that you're there to support and love him—you don't have to try to be his therapist.

This book begins with an overview of major depression and bipolar disorder and gives you background information to better understand what you're dealing with. It discusses the common symptoms of depression and the elevated mood of bipolar disorder using an easy-to-read table. The first chapter also contains a section on the unique features of depression in adolescents, men, women, older persons, and those with other medical illnesses. It includes a description of metabolic syndrome, a condition marked by abdominal obesity, high blood pressure, borderline diabetes, and high fats in the blood, which is closely linked with mood disorders, its medications, and the related disruption in sleep. Metabolic syndrome is not only a side effect of depression treatment but is considered a comorbid condition. Treatment-resistant depression, anxiety, and a Mood Chart to track one's symptoms all follow in this chapter, which concludes with a discussion on stigma.

Chapter 2 explores signs of depression to look for. This includes variations in your family member's or friend's general appearance, vital senses (sleep habits, appetite), and attitude toward herself. I then describe what goes into diagnosing a mood disorder—the emotional and physical changes a clinician looks for. As there are no blood tests, scans, or X-rays to assist the provider, a clinician must rely on observing the patient.

In chapter 3, I review the lifestyle interventions that a person can use to manage her mood disorder. These are things that she has control over, such as accepting her illness and following the Basics of Mental Health (taking medications as prescribed, regular sleep, diet and nutrition, daily physical exercise, having a routine and structure to the day, and avoiding isolation).

Chapter 4 offers a discussion on finding professional help, the different types of mental help providers and treatments available, and shared decision making. You'll learn how to determine when professional help is necessary. This chapter also shows how to choose a mental health provider who is a good fit for your family member and helps you realize what to expect afterward. It concludes with a section on what to do when someone refuses treatment to help you understand the problem and know what steps to take if this occurs.

Chapter 5 offers information on paying for mental health treatment, health insurance coverage options, and what to do when your loved one cannot afford treatment.

In Chapter 6, I discuss how caring for someone who has a mood disorder is different from caring for someone who has other types of medical problems and has unique challenges.

Chapter 7 teaches some support skills and communication strategies uniquely helpful to caregivers of a person who has depression. It covers active listening and the empathic response. It offers concrete examples of what you might say and how you might handle certain situations.

In chapter 8, Helpful Approaches, I present useful suggestions for improving daily interactions with someone who has depression. These include treating him normally and not as a "sick" person, providing hope, having realistic expectations, confronting negative thoughts, knowing when to seek professional help, setting boundaries, and being familiar with the basic guidelines for promoting mental health.

In chapter 9, What You Can Do Now, you will learn to respond effectively to any of the nine main symptoms of depression listed in the *Diagnostic and Statistical Manual of Mental Disorders* (*DSM-5*), the standard diagnostic manual in psychiatry.

Chapter 10 offers valuable advice when you suspect someone is suicidal. It contains the risk factors and warning signs for suicide, as well as what to do if you fear someone is close to self-harm.

Chapter 11 offers a review of combined mood disorders and substance abuse called dual diagnosis. This combination is fairly common as people attempt to self-treat their emotional pain.

Then, in chapter 12, I cover information for parents of an adolescent/teenager or twenty-something. This section includes risk factors unique to this group, symptoms, treatment, school issues, and communication. It concludes with a discussion of and tips for teens and young adults who have a parent affected by depression or bipolar disorder.

Chapter 13 covers the use of technology in mental health, from computers to social media, and in what situations it can be helpful.

Chapter 14, on depression in the senior population, contains specific risk factors in the elderly, symptoms, treatment, and resources for care.

Chapter 15 describes what recovery looks like and the process of recovery in mental health. It then continues on with a discussion of psychological well-being.

Chapter 16, Anticipating Recovery: Skills to Have in Place, suggests how you can foster resilience in someone who has depression or bipolar disorder. *Resilience* is the ability to adapt well during adversity and the capacity to bounce back after difficult times, including from an illness like a mood disorder. Depression is a relapsing and remitting illness that often challenges a person tremendously. Weathering the difficulties will likely decrease the intensity of episodes and often improve your family member's or friend's quality of life.

Chapter 17, Caring for the Caregivers, focuses on you. I first discuss how depression in the family affects all members. Other topics include maintaining your own physical, emotional, and family health and pacing yourself. This is essential to functioning well in a helper role.

Chapter 18 summarizes the dos and don'ts for caregivers in a table for comparison and easy reference, with some suggested language. Following a closing chapter that brings concepts together are a list of useful resources and a glossary of terms. Finally, the appendixes include a list of commonly used medications and what goes into a Psychiatric Advance Directive.

Now we're going to look at who gets depression and bipolar disorder and how it affects the person and his family and friends and what we can do and say, as family members and friends, to help the person get better. We'll begin with the symptoms of depression and how they vary among people.

To the Reader: I understand that you may be dealing with your spouse, significant other, adult or adolescent child, sister or brother, parent, aunt, uncle, grandparent, cousin, or close friend who has depression or bipolar disorder. The language can get rather cumbersome, and it's hard to choose one word that's all-inclusive to represent different family members. For this reason, throughout the book I vary the language, sometimes using a specific relationship and sometimes the grab-bag term "family member or friend." I also vary female and male pronouns, *she* and *he*. In most instances, I mean to include anyone who is affected by depression.

What Are Mood Disorders?

We'll begin our journey with a review of mood disorders. Having background information about depression and bipolar disorder will help you better understand the condition. You'll have an idea of what your family member or friend is experiencing and feeling. That understanding, in turn, will help you say and do what will be most helpful. Many people like you have found this to be true.

Mood disorders are a category of psychiatric conditions that include both major depression and bipolar disorder. Mood disorders involve our state of mind—the part of our inner self that colors and drives our thoughts, feelings, and behaviors. They are biologically based, treatable illnesses that affect all aspects of our lives.

Normally, our mood changes over time and across a broad range of emotions. It can be described using any number of words: *up, down, neutral, happy, sad,* and others. When we're depressed, our mood is persistently very down, and our mental and physical functioning is not as sharp as usual. We don't think as clearly, organize ourselves, or do things as well as before. A negative mood may creep up silently or be related to external or internal events in our lives. *External events* are things that happen to us or around us. A job loss, a relationship breakup, or a visit with a controlling parent are examples of negative external events. *Internal events* include thoughts and feelings inside us, like believing we are unlovable or undesirable.

External and internal events can act as triggers to cause a change in our mood. *Triggers* are events or circumstances that may cause a person distress and increase his depression symptoms. Common triggers include stressful life events both positive (a birth or moving to a new home) and negative (a death or a divorce), conflicts, interpersonal stress, changes in sleep, or substance abuse. Sometimes we cannot identify the trigger that happens before an episode of depression. A dark mood may come on gradually, or it may feel rather sudden after a period of subtle life events.

Each person has his own set of unique triggers. It's helpful for you to become familiar with those events that cause your family member distress.

When you see a trigger affecting him now or coming up in the future, try to make sure he is receiving treatment, taking his medications, managing life's stressors, seeing his mental health professional, and following the Basics of Mental Health (discussed in chapter 3).

MAJOR DEPRESSION

Major depression is also called *depression, major depressive disorder*, or *unipolar depression*. The symptoms of major depression are broad; they negatively affect your family member's or friend's thoughts, feelings, behaviors, physical self, interests, activities, and relationships. A person who has depression often has difficulty with basic everyday functioning, doing things for himself, or concentrating and making decisions. These are symptoms of the illness and are not signs of laziness. They are not intentional.

You may be familiar with the image of a depressed person feeling sad and losing interest in activities. We all feel a little sad at times, but that sadness is different; it is not depression. Sometimes it's hard to tell the difference. Rather, depression is a biologically based medical condition whose symptoms run deeper and last longer than you might expect. Your family member or friend may not feel well or like himself at the start of his illness but may be able to carry on with his usual daily activities. For example, at first he may wake up and get dressed and go through the motions of his day, without much interest or energy. He may feel it's a bit of a struggle to accomplish all the tasks he used to do; the flavor for life has left him. He might not fully understand what is happening to him. The person who has depression is often the last one to realize what is going on. He may deny that he's even experiencing depression. Over time, these symptoms may progress and become more pronounced and interfere with his basic functioning.

> Depression is a biologically based illness of the mind and body with symptoms that last two weeks or longer.

The American Psychiatric Association's *Diagnostic and Statistical Manual of Mental Disorders* (DSM-5) describes depression and gives us a standard way to make the diagnosis. It states that a person must have at least five of the following nine symptoms, lasting two weeks or longer (at least one of the five symptoms must be either persistent sadness or loss of interest) to be diagnosed with depression:

- Persistent sadness, hopelessness, or irritability
- Loss of enjoyment and interest in activities that used to be pleasurable (called anhedonia)
- Loss of appetite or increased appetite, unintentional weight loss due to lack of interest in food; or unintentional weight gain
- Trouble falling asleep or staying asleep, light sleep, sleeping too much or too little, or waking up earlier than necessary
- Feelings of physical agitation or restlessness or of being physically slowed down
- Fatigue or loss of energy for no reason
- Feelings of worthlessness or guilt without foundation
- Decreased ability to focus and concentrate or read
- Recurrent thoughts of death or suicide with or without a plan, or a suicide attempt

Each person may have a different combination of these symptoms—we are not all alike in our illness. Sometimes it can take a long time and become frustrating to find the most effective treatment for each person's unique set of symptoms.

What does it feel like for your family member who has depression? Depression is not just "feeling blue" or mopey for a day or two. It is different from grief, which has a focus, a beginning, and an end. Rather, for many people, depression is a period of deep despair. They see no end in sight, no hope for their future, and no possibility of relief from their fatigue and suffering. They often feel both physical and emotional pain and cannot participate in life. A person who has depression sees only the dark, negative side of the world. He experiences life in a distorted way, with a negative view of himself, his future, and the world. At times, he may feel irritable and take it out on those around him, starting arguments about little things. This is not intentional. He may withdraw from life, friends, and activities. He may lose friends. Communication is often a major effort when depressed.

Your family member may lose interest in the things around him, stop enjoying his past interests, and feel little motivation to participate in life. Sleep and appetite may be markedly affected. He may not sleep except in short naps, or he may sleep too much. Food may be tasteless, or he may binge on junk food as an easy way to ease his pain. Fatigue frequently sets in and compounds the mood symptoms.

Focus and concentration are a challenge to many people who have depression, and his thinking may slow down or become disorganized. This can make work and school difficult and frustrating, particularly for someone used to functioning at a high level. Projects and work often pile up, the mail remains unopened, and the household chores get neglected. He may spend hours just staring straight ahead, unable to tackle the task before him. Some people think about death to relieve their emotional pain. To give you an idea of the type of depression symptoms your family member or friend may have, look over table 1.1. It shows you the range of thoughts, feelings, and behaviors that characterize this illness.

Depression affects everyone in the household.

Depression can be very rough on a family, especially the primary support person. The fluctuating moods of your family member who has depression may add to the stress of a busy household. This can affect everyone around him. It requires time and patience on your part to understand what is going on at the moment, to know whether something has triggered an episode, and to decide how best to respond. You may have many emotions yourself, such as frustration, anger, or guilt. You must be careful to attend to your own and other family members' needs as well and avoid burnout. For more on this topic, refer to chapter 17, Caring for the Caregivers.

Depression and Bipolar Symptoms Can Vary

Mood disorders are most often a *relapsing* and *remitting* illness. This means that it can come and go over time. That is often very frustrating for you and your family member or friend. Depression and manic symptoms come in episodes that may last from several weeks to several months or longer. Each episode can vary in the length of time it lasts and how deep (intense or severe) it is. Examples of the ranges of depression symptom intensity are found in table 1.2. The intervals between episodes of depression or mania also vary. Many people have repeat episodes of depression and may feel and function well in between. Others have a few leftover symptoms in the intervals between episodes, called residual symptoms. The pattern of episodes is unique to each person.

You can better understand your family member's or friend's pattern of depression or bipolar disorder by having him record his moods each day on a Mood Chart (see table 1.6 on pages 31 and 32). This may help him connect his depression symptoms to life events or changes in medications. It is also a good way to follow his progress and response to treatment. Sharing this information with his treatment providers can help them make sound treatment decisions. It can also provide a basis of discussion in therapy sessions.

TABLE 1.1. Symptoms of Depression

NEGATIVE THOUGHTS

- ☐ I deserve this.
- ☐ I'm being punished.
- ☐ It's all my fault.
- ☐ I can't make decisions.
- ☐ I can't remember anything.
- ☐ Nothing good will ever happen.
- ☐ Things will never get better.
- ☐ I never do anything right.
- ☐ I'm not as good as everyone else.

- ☐ Nobody will ever care about me.
- ☐ I'm worthless.
- ☐ People are against me.
- ☐ I should be _____ by now.
- ☐ I've wasted my (life, education, opportunities).
- ☐ There is no hope for me.
- ☐ I think about dying or suicide a lot.

FEELINGS

- ☐ I feel sad for no reason.
- ☐ I don't feel good even if good things happen.
- ☐ I feel worthless.
- ☐ I feel bad; inferior to other people.
- ☐ I feel guilty about everything.

- ☐ I feel easily annoyed or irritated.
- ☐ I fear that something terrible will happen.
- ☐ I feel tired all the time.
- ☐ I'm not interested in anything.
- ☐ I'm not interested in sex.

BEHAVIORS

- ☐ I cry a lot for no reason.
- ☐ I sleep too much.
- ☐ I sleep too little.
- ☐ I eat too much.
- ☐ I eat very little.
- ☐ I drink too much alcohol.
- ☐ I've recently gained a lot of weight.
- ☐ I recently lost a lot of weight without trying.
- ☐ I stay in bed or on the couch all day.
- ☐ Sometimes I don't take a shower, wash my hair, or shave.
- ☐ I have trouble starting or finishing projects.
- ☐ I avoid people and isolate myself.
- ☐ I don't return telephone calls.
- ☐ I've stopped my previous activities and hobbies.

- ☐ I've stopped exercising.
- ☐ I argue and fight with people for no reason.
- ☐ I'm fidgety and restless.
- ☐ I move or speak slowly.
- ☐ I have trouble concentrating.
- ☐ I have difficulty reading the newspaper or following shows on television.
- ☐ I can't keep track of my thoughts to have a conversation.
- ☐ My house is more disorganized than usual.
- ☐ I forget to pay bills.
- ☐ I forget to do or don't do laundry or other household duties.
- ☐ I call in sick to work or school a lot.

Source: Susan J. Noonan, *Managing Your Depression: What You Can Do to Feel Better* (Johns Hopkins University Press, 2013), 43.

TABLE 1.2. Intensity of Depression Symptoms

SYMPTOMS OF DEPRESSION	MILD	MODERATE	SEVERE
Depressed mood, hopelessness, or irritability	Is dispirited but still functioning	Feels sad and unhappy most of time or irritable	Looks and feels totally miserable; unable to function
Diminished interest or pleasure in things	Has reduced interest in things	Has greater loss of interest or pleasure	Is unable to feel any emotion or pleasure
Weight loss or gain OR increased or decreased appetite	Has mild loss of taste	Lost or gained 2–5 lb. unintentionally; no appetite	Lost or gained 5 lb. or more unintentionally; needs persuasion to eat
Sleeping too much OR too little	Has slight difficulty falling asleep or sleeps lightly	Has several awakenings interrupting sleep (~2 hrs.)	Sleeps 2–3 hrs. per night OR over 10 hrs. total
Physical restlessness OR slowing down	Has difficulty starting activities	Finds activities are carried out with great effort	Is unable to do anything without help OR is pacing, restless
Fatigue or loss of energy nearly every day	Has difficulty starting activities	Finds activities are carried out with great effort	Is unable to do anything without help
Feelings of worthlessness or guilt	Occasionally feels worthless	Frequently feels worthless or guilty	Has frequent and intrusive thoughts of worthlessness
Diminished ability to think or concentrate; make decisions	Has occasional and mild episodes	Has frequent and marked episodes	Has this every day and it's intrusive; is unable to read or converse normally
Recurrent thoughts of death or suicide, a plan, or a suicide attempt	Has fleeting thoughts of suicide	Has common thoughts but no specific suicide plans or intention	Has explicit plans for suicide

Relapse and Recurrence

This isn't what you want to hear, I know, but depression and bipolar disorder are not always onetime experiences. Even those who are successfully treated and recover from an episode many have a repeat episode, called a *relapse* or *recurrence*. A relapse is the return of full depressive symptoms after *partial recovery* from an episode. A recurrence is the return of full depressive symptoms following a *full recovery* from an episode (table 1.3).

Sixty percent of those who have had one episode of depression and recover will have a second one at some time in their life. Seventy percent of those with two episodes will experience a third, and 90 percent of those with three episodes will have a fourth. Don't be disheartened. Depression is treatable and the symptoms can be managed. *Cognitive Behavioral Therapy* (CBT), a type of talk therapy that addresses the connection between our thoughts, feelings, and behaviors, and *Mindfulness-based CBT* can decrease the chance of relapse and recurrence.

TABLE 1.3 **Definitions of Antidepressant Treatment Responses**	
RESPONSE	Partial improvement in symptoms and at least a 50% reduction in depression severity as measured by standardized rating questionnaires
REMISSION	Depressive symptoms completely cleared
RELAPSE	Return of full depressive symptoms after partial recovery from an episode
RECURRENCE	Return of full depressive symptoms following full recovery from an episode

Source: Adapted from A. A. Nierenberg and L. M. DeCecco, "Definitions of Antidepressant Treatment Response, Remission, Nonresponse, Partial Response, and Other Relevant Outcomes: A Focus on Treatment-Resistant Depression," *Journal of Clinical Psychiatry* 62, suppl. 16 (2001): 15–19.

The Theory of Depression

Imagine the brain as a network of brain cells (called *neurons*) bathed in special chemicals that help the cells communicate with each other, sending messages from cell to cell. One long-held view is that depression disrupts these chemicals, called *neurotransmitters*, found in the part of the brain that regulates emotions and behavior. The chemical disruption is thought to happen when certain life events occur in a susceptible person.

Another theory involves the interaction of our genes and the events in our life (our environment) that shape the complex network of cells in our brain. This is called the *gene × environment* theory. Our *environment* includes the people, thoughts, and events that occur around us, both inside and outside our bodies. This could be inside or outside stress, an illness, or a traumatic event. Examples of stressful life events include a major loss or death, marriage or divorce, a new job or loss of a job, chronic stress, hormonal changes (such as during perimenopause or postpartum), medical illness, substance abuse, sleep disorders, and positive events like the birth of a baby or moving to a new home.

A *gene* is a precise arrangement of molecules (a sequence of DNA) that makes up the chromosomes in our cells. Genes are inherited from each of our parents. They direct the body to make certain proteins that control our normal bodily functions, including those of our brain. Scientists have found genes associated with certain disease conditions, including some psychiatric illnesses such as schizophrenia, bipolar disorder, and depression. A study by Hyde and associates (2016) identified 15 genes linked to major depression in persons of European descent. And now over 60 genes associated with a susceptibility to bipolar disorder have been identified. These findings may help us to better understand these illnesses and to design new interventions and treatments in the future.

> Depression involves the complex interaction of our genes with events in our environment.

The *gene × environment* theory of depression is thought to work in this way. The brain is sensitive to stressful and traumatic events during vulnerable periods in our life. Negative stimulation, such as stress or illness, changes the action of certain genes. When this happens, it affects the shape of the network of cells in our brain (the *neural network*) and its functioning. If stress or illness changes gene activity during a vulnerable period, the genes and our brains do not work as well. When that happens during a vulnerable period, it affects our feelings, thoughts, and behaviors, and the result is depression. Depression is not entirely genetic and not entirely related to life experiences. It requires a "perfect storm" of both coming together at a time when the person is vulnerable. The combination of events (stressors) in one's environment along with a genetic susceptibility to depression, occurring in a person who is in a vulnerable period of their life, can lead to an episode of depression. Since we can all experience a variety of losses and stressors in our life, there are many ways that this can happen.

Your loved one may have genetic factors that make him more likely to suffer from depression, but this *does not guarantee* that he will have the illness. If a person is genetically prone to depression, he may not have an episode unless he also experiences certain stressful life events. These experiences are thought to affect the genes that regulate our brain functioning.

Depression often runs in families, which supports the idea of a genetic basis for the illness. This was seen in research studies of depression in twins, who by definition share some of the same genetic material. The research showed that first-degree relatives of those who have major depression have an increased risk of depression in part due to shared genes, separate from shared family experiences. These results provide support for the inherited (genetic) theory of depression.

The exciting news is that understanding how genes work in mood disorders will allow researchers to design new treatment interventions. In the future, some of these may be targeted to a person's specific combination of symptoms or subtype of depression.

> Understanding how genes work in depression will allow us to design new treatment interventions.

Scientists have proposed other recent, exciting theories of depression. One cutting-edge theory of depression in 2020 regards mood disorders as an *inflammatory process*. An illness such as depression would then involve the activation of a cascade of chemical events in the body's immune system. Supporting the theory of an inflammatory process, psychiatrists have seen that minocycline, an antibiotic, has successfully treated depression in certain people. Research scientists are working hard to further our understanding of the inflammatory process and its relationship to mental illness, with the hopes of designing improved and targeted treatments in the future. Another lesser known theory of depression involves a dysfunction of the little organelle inside of our cells that produces energy, called the mitochondria. It may be a way to explain the fatigue and physical symptoms of depression. Evidence on this connection is early yet has potential promise.

DEPRESSION BY AGE, SEX, OR ILLNESS

Depression in Women

In women, mood disorders and anxiety peak in adolescence and early adulthood. Females are at much greater risk than males and have twice the lifetime rates of depression and most anxiety disorders. Puberty, the menstrual cycle, pregnancy, and the transition to menopause are triggers for the onset, recurrence, and worsening of mood disorders and anxiety. This suggests hormonal involvement.

The influence of reproductive hormones on mood in a woman occurs in addition to psychosocial burdens and stressors of life events. Balancing work and family, maintaining households and finances, caring for elderly parents, single parenting, and experiencing poverty, limited social support, or other social and health problems can impact a mood disorder. When a woman who has depression is a wife, a mother, or pregnant, her illness can affect the entire family. Children growing up in a household where the mother has depression or bipolar disorder may experience a variety of emotional problems themselves, as their maternal-child bonding is affected, and they are quick to pick up on the moods and behaviors of their parents. A spouse or significant other can also feel the effects of maternal depression and can experience symptoms of postpartum depression.

> **Some women have an abnormal response to the cyclic changes in normal reproductive hormones, which can lead to depression.**

Females undergo changes in their reproductive hormones during their growth and development, which can affect brain function and mood disorders. The amount of estrogen and progesterone shifts throughout a woman's life, and each month during her reproductive years (teens to menopause) a woman's level of these hormones normally goes up and down in a characteristic cyclic pattern.

Some women are considered vulnerable to changes in the body's level of *estrogen* and *progesterone*, the reproductive hormones produced primarily in the ovaries. Estrogen is thought to have an effect on certain neurotransmitters (brain chemicals like serotonin and noradrenaline involved in mood regulation) that may contribute to the onset of depressive symptoms in some women. During puberty, the start of ovarian functioning and cycling, a girl's estrogen levels rise significantly and this parallels with the onset and increased rates of depression in this age group.

Rapid change occurs in reproductive hormones during the last week of the menstrual cycle, during the postpartum period, and during the transition to menopause. It is thought that *some* women are vulnerable to and have an abnormal response to these normal reproductive hormone changes and fluctuations, leading to mood disorders and depression. This results in periods of sadness, irritability, depressed mood, anxiety, and other emotional and physical symptoms like fluid retention and fatigue.

If this experience happens right before the menstrual period, it is called *premenstrual syndrome*, or PMS. PMS refers to a pattern of physical, emotional, and behavioral symptoms that occur one to two weeks before the menstrual period and end when the period begins. PMS is thought to be related to an increased reactivity to the elevated levels of progesterone at this time. It affects approximately 20 to 25 percent of women, or more. Symptoms of PMS include anger, anxiety, depression, irritability, poor concentration, bloating, breast tenderness, fatigue, and muscle aches.

Premenstrual dysphoric disorder (PMDD), a more severe form of PMS, is associated with significant distress and interferes with functioning and quality of life. Irritability is its hallmark symptom. PMDD affects approximately 5 percent of women. A type of antidepressant called selective serotonin reuptake inhibitors, or SSRIs, are considered first-line treatment for PMDD; lifestyle modifications, such as healthy diet and exercise, may also help.

A current theory about the cause of PMS/PMDD is that it may be an abnormal response to the normal fluctuations of hormones in some women, who have different sensitivity to normal changes in estrogen and progesterone. Another theory has recently linked PMDD to a set of genes on our chromosomes. It shows that women who experience PMDD have a basic difference in the way their cells respond to reproductive hormones. The evidence of a genetic link to PMDD also offers the potential for future treatment options in this and other reproductive hormone–related mood disorders.

Mood disorder symptoms can also worsen right before a woman's menstrual period in a pattern that is different from PMDD. This occurs in women who have an underlying mood disorder and is called *premenstrual exacerbation*, or *PME*. The difference is that the mood symptoms in PME do not go away when menses begins (as happens in PMDD), and symptoms last throughout the entire menstrual cycle. Approximately 40 percent of women who are screened for PMDD have an underlying mood disorder with PME. To make the diagnosis and tell the difference, use a Mood Chart for at least two months, tracking the days of the month of her menstrual period and other symptoms (see table 1.6 on page 32).

> Postpartum depression occurs in 10 to 15 percent of women.

Women may also experience *depression* during pregnancy or after childbirth, when it's called postpartum depression. Postpartum depression is more than the "baby blues," which peak two to five days after delivery and can last two weeks. Baby blues typically include tearfulness, sadness, quickly varying moods, irritability and anxiety but does not seriously impair functioning or include psychotic symptoms (loss of reality). Postpartum depression occurs in 10 to 15 percent of women. It has more severe symptoms and impairs functioning and the infant-mother attachment (bonding). During pregnancy, women are exposed to very high levels of hormones made by the placenta. Postpartum depression is related to a rapid shift in these hormones after giving birth.

Symptoms of postpartum depression may be mild, with bouts of sadness and tearfulness, or deep and extreme.

Women who experience postpartum depression fall into three groups: (1) one-fourth have had chronic depression before pregnancy, (2) one-third have the onset of depression during pregnancy, and (3) slightly more than one-third have the onset of depression in the period after giving birth (postpartum). Women who have a history of depression are three times more likely to experience postpartum depression; this rate is even higher for those who experience depression during pregnancy. Untreated depression during pregnancy increases the chance of postpartum depression. Untreated postpartum depression affects the health of the woman, infant, and rest of the family.

A very serious symptom of postpartum depression is *postpartum psychosis*, which occurs in one to two per 1,000 births and usually begins within the first few days after delivery. Its hallmarks are loss of touch with reality, delusions (fixed false beliefs), hallucinations, bizarre behavior, confusion, and disorganized thinking, accompanied by depression or an elevated mood. Postpartum psychosis is a psychiatric emergency.

Some women going through *menopause* may have episodes of depression. During menopause, the body naturally slows its reproductive hormone cycles, and a woman stops having menstrual periods. This is associated with changes in estrogen levels and a decline in the functioning of her ovaries, which causes her to make less estrogen (or *estradiol*). This may trigger depression in some vulnerable women. Symptoms can include fatigue, trouble sleeping, difficulty with concentration and remembering small details, hot flashes, night sweats, and mood shifts.

Depression at this time is called *perimenopausal*, *menopausal*, or *postmenopausal* depression. *Perimenopause* begins three to five years before menopause, when hormone production becomes erratic and overall estrogen levels begin to slowly drop. It is considered the transition phase to menopause. Mood disorders may occur during this time; there is a four to six times greater risk of depression in women who have had a history of major depression, and a two to three times greater risk in those with no history. *Menopause* begins, on average, at age 47 and lasts four to eight years. *Postmenopause* occurs when a woman's monthly periods finally stop. Researchers have learned that the risk of experiencing depression is greater for women during and immediately after the transition to menopause, a highly vulnerable time period than when they are premenopausal. This is true whether she has ever had a prior episode of depression. Episodes of depression can become less frequent and may sometimes disappear once a woman passes through menopause. Interestingly, after menopause the rates of depression in women are lower, closer to those seen in men.

Women can be at greater risk for depression during menopause if they have a prior history of depression, social stressors, health conditions with chronic medical problems, and poor social support. Also, women whose sleep has been affected by severe hot flashes (vasomotor symptoms) and women who seem to have wider hormone fluctuations may experience depression more often.

> A decline in ovarian function and estrogen levels may trigger depression in some women.

It is thought that menopausal vasomotor symptoms (hot flashes and night sweats causing frequent awakenings) are triggered by a fall in estrogen and other reproductive (sex) hormones circulating in the bloodstream; these can negatively affect sleep, mood, and the quality of life. Several preliminary research studies have shown that an antagonist to the brain hormone NKB-neurokinin 3 receptor may be related to estrogen deficiency hot flashes (NKB-neurokinin is found in the hypothalamus in the brain, an area that regulates body temperature, sleep, appetite, and emotional responses and other things). A 2020 research study (Tower 2020) reported that the drug NT-814 (a dual antagonist to neurokinin 1 and 3 receptor) showed rapid and marked improvement in hot flashes and interrupted sleep due to night sweats and was well tolerated. This is exciting news; it suggests a new nonhormonal approach to the management of vasomotor symptoms in menopausal women. Further research is pending.

To find a potential association between hormone levels and your loved one's depression, encourage her to use the Mood Chart (table 1.6) to track her moods. Make sure that she includes the days of her menstrual cycle and other important events, such as the birth of a child, in the notes section on the chart. Then she can share the completed chart with her mental health provider.

You might wonder, Why not just treat a woman with estrogen supplements? Researchers have looked at this; while there are not very many strong scientific studies (RCTs, or randomized controlled trials) and data are limited, they have learned the following. In women who are not depressed, there is no scientific evidence that shows the benefit of estrogen supplements on mood. Estrogen does not treat or prevent depression in those who are not already depressed. In women who are currently depressed, estrogen use resulted in significant improvement in mood in those who are in perimenopause. This is considered equivalent to the effect seen with classic antidepressant medications in depressed perimenopausal women. Mood improvement was not associated with improvement in nighttime hot flashes or sleep. Estrogen has also been used effectively as an augmentation, or additional therapy, to antidepressant medications. However, the same hormone formulation (17-B estradiol skin patch or E2) was not effective in treating major depression in postmenopausal women. This suggests that the transition to menopause, called perimenopause, might be a critical window of opportunity for estrogen treatment in those who are at risk for depression or who have depression. Estrogen therapy, along with its side effects and risks, must be discussed with your provider.

Estrogen use can be helpful in those who have depression and are in perimenopause, the transition to menopause.

The exact relationship between mood and hormones is not fully understood, but research is ongoing. The Massachusetts General Hospital Center for Women's Mental Health website (www.womens mentalhealth.org) is a valuable resource on women and depression. Here, you will find a library of information, a newsletter, and a blog covering up-to-date topics, including depression and PMS and PMDD, perinatal and postpartum depression, fertility and mental health, and menopausal symptoms.

Depression in Men

Some men who experience depression become irritable and agitated, rather than sad, as their major symptom of a mood disorder. Your family member may appear cranky and irritable instead of sad or tearful when depressed. Irritability can lead him to persistently direct angry outbursts or frustration over minor matters toward others. Sometimes, he won't be able to tolerate another person nearby, even if he knows you mean well.

Men who have depression often have more anger attacks, acts of aggression, substance abuse issues, and risk-taking behaviors than women. Some may scream and yell; argue; break things; engage in risky behaviors such as gambling, drinking, or substance abuse; engage in excessive sexual behavior; or work too much as a sign of depression. An agitated depression can be very difficult to treat because your family member's or friend's actions can be unpredictable.

Mental health researchers commonly report that women experience symptoms of depression twice as often as men. In 2016 in the United States, 8.5 percent of adult women and 4.8 percent of adult men had at least one major depressive episode (National Institute of Mental Health 2016). At the same time, 3.1 million adolescents ages 12 to 17, including 19.4 percent of adolescent girls and 6.4 percent of adolescent boys had at least one major depressive episode (National Institute of Mental Health 2016). These differences may be related to issues common to women, including the stress of family and social obligations and hormone fluctuations during puberty, the menstrual cycle, before and after childbirth (as in postpartum depression), and during the transition to menopause.

Many men have been raised to withhold their feelings and not talk about their sadness or emotional pain.

However, some psychiatric providers wonder whether these numbers are accurate. They question whether we are identifying all of the instances of depression in men. It might *look* as if women experience twice the rate of depression as men when perhaps the actual numbers are closer. This is because men may experience different symptoms or fail to report the traditional symptoms of depression, such as sadness, fatigue, loss of interest, sleep, or appetite. Most men may find admitting to sadness or crying socially unacceptable. They are often brought up to withhold their feelings. Men who experience emotional distress may also be more likely to react with anger, aggression, irritability, or self-destructive and risk-taking behavior. They may numb their pain with alcohol, drugs, gambling, or excess work.

In 2013, University of Michigan researchers looked at whether men and women experience depression equally (Martin, Neighbors, and Griffith 2013). They gathered information using a self-report questionnaire of English-speaking adults in the United States. First, they looked at gender differences in depression symptoms using a rating scale. They found that "male specific" symptoms such as anger, aggression, alcohol and substance use, irritability, and risk-taking behavior were more common in men than women.

We may not be identifying all the episodes of depression in men.

Researchers then combined these symptoms with 15 traditional symptoms of depression in a new rating scale. Men and women met the definition for depression in fairly equal numbers when measured using this combined rating scale. The researchers believe that current depression screening, which relies only on traditional symptoms, may fail to include symptoms common to men. As a result, depression in men may be underreported. More studies are needed to understand fully which symptoms accurately identify depression in men and to learn whether men and women experience depression in equal proportions.

There are some limitations to this study. It is a "secondary data analysis" study, which means that it was planned out in advance and information was collected and analyzed after the fact. The authors were able to evaluate most but not all potential symptoms of depression. Also, there were two time frames for answering the study questions ("in your lifetime" and "in the past 30 days"). None of this affects the point of the study for our purpose.

Depression in Adolescents

Depression in adolescents and young adults has been rising. The National Surveys on Drug Use and Health reviewed 172,495 adolescents and 178,755 young adults (18–25 years old) from 2005 to 2014. Their report showed that in 2014 the number of major depression episodes for that 12-month period had increased to 11.3 percent in adolescents and 9.6 percent in young adults.

Irritability and agitation may be the primary feature of depression in your child or adolescent. You may notice a difference in his school or work performance, a loss of friends or a new crowd of friends, or a change in activities he once enjoyed. Your teenager might be more withdrawn and secretive about what she does and where she goes—and with whom. She may become argumentative and fight with you or her siblings.

Your daughter may become tearful and withdrawn, especially around the time of menstruation. Some adolescents may miss days of school or work or take a temporary leave of absence from school. Alcohol, illegal drugs, and reckless driving can become issues. The important thing is that you notice and respond to any unusual changes in your adolescent's typical emotions and behavior. (See chapter 12, For the Parents of a Teen or a Young Adult.)

Anxiety is the most common form of psychiatric illness in children. The combination of depression and anxiety is common, seen in over one-half of children, and it can lead to a more difficult diagnostic assessment, more severe symptoms, and more complicated treatments. These children and adolescents may have more bodily complaints of physical illness (stomachaches, for example, with missed days of school), irritability and agitation, impaired functioning in school and socially during their important developmental years, obsessive thoughts and compulsive behaviors, and increased risk of suicide.

Treating anxiety and depression in adolescence is important because early onset of these conditions increases the risk of depression in adulthood. Early intervention of depression and anxiety in adolescence may decrease the burden of illness in later life.

Depression in the Elderly

Depression can also affect the senior members of your family, and it can be sometimes difficult to determine whether the problem is depression, an extended grief response, or a cognitive decline. Elderly persons often experience health problems and physical impairments that limit their lifestyle, a loss of independence and purpose, and the loss of loved ones, all of which can contribute to depression. This is where the family doctor can be most helpful in sorting out the correct diagnosis. There is a more detailed discussion of this topic in chapter 14.

Depression in Medical Illness

Family members and friends who have certain long-lasting medical problems experience a lot of stress and may be prone to mood disorders. Stress, related to having a chronic illness, can be stuck in overdrive and can change the body and the brain. In some instances, people may lose their lifestyle and purpose in life, their physical activities may be limited, and they might be in pain or in fear of losing their life. These circumstances can affect mood in vulnerable individuals. Here are some examples of how medical problems can affect mood.

When your body makes too much thyroid hormone, mania can be triggered, while too little thyroid can lead to depression. Lack of vitamin B12 in the diet can lead to depression, which is common in the elderly. Up to 50 percent of people who have heart disease or certain types of cancer, such as breast cancer, will also face depression.

Other medical problems are associated with depression:

- Multiple sclerosis
- Parkinson disease
- Alzheimer disease
- Huntington disease
- Stroke
- Certain immune system diseases, such as lupus
- Mononucleosis

In addition, some of the medications used to treat physical medical problems may lead to depression (see table 14.1 on page 184). These include some antimicrobials and antibiotics, heart and blood pressure drugs such as beta-blockers (propranolol, metoprolol, or atenolol), calcium channel blockers (verapamil, nifedipine), digoxin, and methyldopa. Hormones such as anabolic steroids, estrogens (Premarin), prednisone, and birth control pills may contribute to depression, as well as some miscellaneous drugs like clonazepam (Klonopin), cimetidine and ranitidine (Zantac), and narcotic pain medications. Withdrawal from cocaine or amphetamines may also cause depression.

As with depression from other causes, the good news is that depression related to long-term medical problems is treatable. The key is to recognize that depression is happening and to seek professional mental health treatment early on. Some heart centers and oncology departments have mental health professionals on their team, ready to receive referrals from treating physicians.

SYMPTOMS OF ADVANCED DEPRESSION

On occasion a person who has depression or bipolar disorder may have such distorted thoughts that he loses touch with reality. His perception of the world becomes wildly inaccurate. His speech and thoughts are disorganized. These *psychotic features* indicate severe illness. He may experience *hallucinations*, seeing or hearing things that are not actually there. Because these hallucinations may seem real, the concern is that he could act on what he is "told" to do by imagined voices.

He may have paranoid delusions (fixed false beliefs) and believe he is being stalked or followed, that the FBI is tapping his telephone, or that his body organs are decaying inside him. In the mania of bipolar disorder, he might be convinced that he has superhuman powers and can do anything extraordinarily well. It can be both scary and confusing for you to witness these episodes. Any of these features constitute a psychiatric emergency. The person needs immediate evaluation and treatment by a mental health professional.

TREATMENT-RESISTANT DEPRESSION

Have you seen the terms *treatment-resistant depression* or *difficult-to-treat depression* (focused on symptom control and functional improvement)? This implies that, despite trying various medications and treatments, the person has not seen improvement in his depression symptoms or level of functioning. Until recently, it was thought that many people who have difficult-to-treat or treatment-resistant depression have been inadequately treated or undertreated.

Choosing a treatment plan for depression is a complex medical decision requiring an experienced psychiatrist. However, the reality is that many antidepressant medications are prescribed by primary care physicians, often in consultation with a psychiatrist. Primary care physicians may see the early or milder cases of the illness, while a specialist in psychiatry often sees the more complex or prolonged ones. Yet even in the best hands, some people fail to see an improvement in their symptoms or level of functioning after one course of treatment so they get discouraged.

Researchers have learned that many factors may contribute to "treatment resistance": the medication dosage is too low, the medication has not been given a chance to work, or the medication is not tolerated well and so the individual has stopped taking it because of side effects. Perhaps it's not the best choice of drug for his particular type of symptoms. Now new, better-tolerated medications, combined with careful attention to standard psychiatric treatment guidelines by providers, have changed this thinking.

> More than 60 percent of the antidepressant medications are prescribed by a primary care physician, not a psychiatrist.

Currently, psychiatrists see many people who fail to respond (defined as partial improvement in symptoms) or achieve remission (defined as complete relief, free of depression symptoms) after an adequate course of treatment. There is no single definition of or accepted diagnostic criteria for treatment-resistant depression. It may mean failure to improve after one course of an antidepressant of adequate dose and duration, or it may mean failure to respond to three or more courses of antidepressants and other treatments, including talk therapy or electroconvulsive therapy (ECT) over several months or more.

Response to treatment often takes weeks or months, and many people require multiple attempts at treatment before they reach a satisfactory response. Medications are generally helpful in about 60 to 70 percent of people. Only 50 percent of those who have depression respond to a first course of antidepressant treatment, and only 33 percent achieve full remission after a first course. This can all be discouraging for you and your family member. A consultation with an experienced psychiatrist to review medications and other treatment can be quite valuable.

There are three main reasons why antidepressants don't seem to work for some people:

1. *Drug selection and dosing issues.* The "effective" dose for each person will vary with his or her age, gender, weight, physical health, and the other medications. No absolute "correct" dose applies to everyone. Some people metabolize medications at a faster or slower rate than others. In addition, there are many different types of antidepressants; some work better for one subtype of depression symptom than another (atypical, melancholic, or seasonal depression). So, a person may have a treatment failure if he is not on the most effective dose for him. The dose may be too low, taken for too short a period, or cause side effects.

2. *Inaccurate diagnosis.* Sometimes it's difficult to make the correct diagnosis if other issues are going on in the person's life. Or a diagnosis

of bipolar disorder can be mistaken for major depression, particularly if it is the person's first episode and she has not yet had mania or hypomania to indicate bipolar illness. That could lead someone to be wrongly labeled "treatment resistant" or "difficult to treat." Perhaps a person has a different subtype of depression not accurately appreciated by the provider. This matters because the different subtypes respond differently to various antidepressants.

3. *No response despite appropriate treatment type, dose, and duration.* This much smaller group may be experiencing true treatment resistance. Several therapeutic options are available for these individuals.

Medication options for treatment-resistant depression can be (1) to switch to another antidepressant, (2) to augment the antidepressant drug by adding a non-antidepressant drug (such as lithium, atypical antipsychotics, thyroid hormone, herbal products, etc.) to enhance the effects of the antidepressant drug, or (3) to combine different types of antidepressants.

Other treatment options might include psychotherapy or neurostimulation, a method that uses low electrical or magnetic current to stimulate the mood centers of the brain. These can be either noninvasive or invasive therapies. Noninvasive examples include ECT and repetitive transcranial magnetic stimulation. Invasive therapies such as deep brain stimulation require brain surgery and are not considered lightly. Chapter 4 has more information about these therapies. Even when they are under the care of experts, some individuals may still be difficult to treat. Psychiatrists urge the person who has depression not to despair or give up on treatment.

BIPOLAR DISORDER

Bipolar disorder, known as *manic depressive disorder* in the past, is another mood disorder. Like depression, it is a relapsing and remitting illness with a significant impact on daily life. Bipolar disorder is considered a dysregulation of brain cells and is thought to be associated with genes that interfere with the normal functioning of the brain. Scientists have now identified about 60 genes so far. Bipolar disorder is characterized by *manic episodes*, periodic episodes of extreme elevated mood or irritability, alternating with episodes of extreme depression, or *bipolar depression*. These episodes come in cycles; the pattern differs for each person, although there are usually many more episodes of depression. It usually requires continuous long-term treatment.

The symptoms of bipolar depression are similar to major depression; the *DSM-5* diagnostic list is similar to that for major depression. It takes time and the skills of an experienced mental health professional to accurately diagnosis bipolar depression and unipolar (major) depression. Moreover, the treatment for each is very different.

The *DSM-5* states that to be diagnosed with a bipolar manic episode, a person must experience an elevated or irritable mood that impairs functioning and lasts for at least one week, as well as at least three of the following symptoms:

- Inflated sense of self or grandiosity
- Increased physical and mental activity and agitated body movements (*psychomotor agitation*)
- Decreased need for sleep
- Racing thoughts
- Easily distracted with poor concentration
- Pressured speech—more talkative than usual (rapid, loud, nonstop talking)
- Irritability
- High-risk behaviors (excessive spending, impulsive sexual behavior, etc.)

The different types of bipolar disorder—*bipolar I*, *bipolar II*, *bipolar spectrum*, and *mixed states*—cross a spectrum of these symptoms. The bipolar type depends on the depth and length of time the elevated mood symptoms last.

Bipolar type	Elevated mood	Depressed mood
Bipolar I	Manic episodes	Depressive episodes
Bipolar II	Hypomanic episodes	(Prolonged) depressive episodes
Bipolar spectrum	Symptoms in between	
Mixed state	Combination of mania (or hypomania) and depression at same time	

A person who has bipolar I typically has manic episodes and depressive episodes. People who have bipolar II experience hypomanic episodes and prolonged depressive episodes. The symptoms of bipolar spectrum fall somewhere in between. A *manic episode* is as described earlier. A *hypomanic episode* is less intense and shorter in length, and *mixed states* are a combination of mania (or hypomania) and depression symptoms that happen at the same time. Examples of symptoms of an elevated mood are presented in table 1.4.

A study following those who have bipolar disorder for 12 years found that those who have bipolar I had symptoms about 50 percent of the time, with depression about one-third of the time, mania about 10 percent of the time, and mixed symptoms about 6 percent of the time.

What does it feel like for your family member or friend who has bipolar disorder? Most find it very difficult to go through the different phases of mania, hypomania, depression, or a mixed state. Bipolar depression is similar to major depression. During this time, he may withdraw from friends and family. He may feel too irritable to be around people. Problems with concentration and focus can affect his work or school. Symptoms of fatigue, sadness, loss of interest, loss of appetite, and sleep disturbances are common. Negative thinking dominates in many people during the depressed phase.

At the other extreme, a manic or hypomanic episode is often described as having a storm inside one's head. Characteristically, when a person is manic, his thoughts and speech race from idea to idea without completing a thought. Your family member or friend might be too disorganized and distracted to function well but fails to realize it. In fact, like many in the manic phase, he may believe he can do anything—and do it extraordinarily well. This is not actually the case.

Your family member or friend may feel energized, with little or no need for sleep. He might engage in impulsive, high-risk behaviors, such as compulsive shopping and spending money, excessive drinking, illegal drug use, reckless driving, or extreme sexual behavior. His actions could potentially lead to poor social, financial, and business decisions. They affect the person with bipolar disorder and everyone around him.

MOOD CHART

A Mood Chart is a way for your family member to track her symptoms over time instead of trying to remember the details of what each day was like. It's easy to use. Encourage your family member or friend who has a mood disorder to use the Mood Chart every day for a month to start and share it with her mental health provider. All she needs to do is check a box that best describes her mood that day. For example, she might choose a depressed mood that she estimates to be *severe*, *moderate*, or *mild* (see table 1.2). Have her make the best guess. It doesn't have to be exact. A sample completed Mood Chart is provided in table 1.5 on page 31.

TABLE 1.4. Symptoms of Elevated Mood

ELEVATED THOUGHTS

- ☐ I have special abilities.
- ☐ I have a lot of good ideas.
- ☐ My thoughts are really great.
- ☐ Many people are interested in me and my ideas.
- ☐ Many people are against me.
- ☐ I get very focused on a project or cause.
- ☐ My thoughts jump around quickly from one topic to another.
- ☐ Other people say they can't follow what I'm saying.
- ☐ The rest of the world is too slow.
- ☐ It takes others a really long time to do things.

FEELINGS

- ☐ I feel good even when bad things happen.
- ☐ I feel happy without reason.
- ☐ I'm very self-confident.
- ☐ I feel like I have lots of energy even when I get less sleep than usual.
- ☐ I feel optimistic about everything.
- ☐ I feel great, on top of the world.
- ☐ I feel that everything will go my way.
- ☐ I feel that nothing bad can happen to me.
- ☐ I feel that I'm easily annoyed or irritated.
- ☐ I'm very impatient.
- ☐ I feel more interested in sex than usual.

BEHAVIORS

- ☐ I sleep less than usual but don't feel tired.
- ☐ I laugh a lot or for no reason.
- ☐ I'm more talkative than usual.
- ☐ I'm fidgety, restless, and I pace.
- ☐ I have trouble concentrating.
- ☐ I'm easily distracted.
- ☐ I start lots of new projects and activities.
- ☐ I've increased my activities, work, and hobbies.
- ☐ I don't finish projects before starting new ones.
- ☐ I'm much more sociable than usual.
- ☐ I make more phone calls than usual.
- ☐ I spend money and go on shopping sprees.
- ☐ I make impulsive decisions.
- ☐ I tip excessively and gamble.
- ☐ I take more risks than usual.
- ☐ I do more risky or dangerous activities.
- ☐ I start arguments or fights for no reason.
- ☐ I drive fast.
- ☐ I've increased my use of alcohol or drugs.
- ☐ I dress flashier than usual.
- ☐ My handwriting has gotten larger and messier.

Source: Susan J. Noonan, *Managing Your Depression: What You Can Do to Feel Better* (Johns Hopkins University Press, 2013), 44.

The Mood Chart may help your family member or friend track fluctuations in his illness and identify patterns in his mood over a month's time. It is a better reflection of his illness than trying to remember these details during a doctor's or therapist's appointment. The "Notes" column on the Mood Chart is meant to record anything that may have affected his mood that day, such as a change in medications or a stressful event. Women might record hormonal changes or a menstrual period. A blank Mood Chart is provided as table 1.6 on page 32.

As you can see after filling in the Mood Chart, the daily course of depression typically fluctuates. In addition, each of your family member's or friend's symptoms can separately vary in how deep or severe it feels. This means he could experience a range of feelings or behaviors for each particular symptom.

For example, if he has a "depressed mood or irritability," he could feel anywhere from slightly blue to overwhelmingly down, devastated and unable to function, or somewhere in between. Many people find this kind of variation to be true. Or he could either have a slight to moderate "loss of appetite" or perhaps lose 10 pounds over two weeks because he lacks all interest in food. For variations within each symptom of depression refer to table 1.1.

Why is this important? The variations in symptoms and their pattern are unique to every person and are unpredictable. Your friend's or family member's doctors will be helped greatly in deciding on the best course of treatment if they can see his symptom variation.

MOOD DISORDERS AND METABOLIC SYNDROME

Metabolic syndrome is a physical health condition that is often seen in those who have mental illness, particularly bipolar disorder and schizophrenia. It can be found in those who have major depression, particularly if your family member takes certain antidepressants or antipsychotic medications or has signs of general inflammation confirmed by a blood test. Metabolic syndrome is also related to lack of sleep and disrupted sleep patterns, something that is common in mood disorders. In 2014, C. D. Rethorst and other researchers at the University of Texas at Dallas studied a national health survey and found metabolic syndrome in just over 41 percent of people who have depression.

Metabolic syndrome is a physiologic problem of obesity and weight gain primarily in the belly (abdomen), increased lipids (fats) in the blood, high

DAY	DEPRESSED			NEUTRAL	ELEVATED MOOD			NOTES
	severe	moderate	mild	neutral	mild	moderate	severe	
1	✓							
2	✓							
3		✓						Argument with father
4		✓						
5		✓						
6		✓						
7	✓							
8	✓							
9	✓							Added new medication
10		✓						
11		✓						
12		✓						
13			✓					
14			✓					
15			✓					
16		✓						
17			✓					
18			✓					
19				✓				
20				✓				
21			✓					
22								
23								
24								
25								
26								
27								
28								
29								
30								
31								

TABLE 1.5. **Sample Completed Mood Chart**

Source: Susan J. Noonan, *Managing Your Depression: What You Can Do to Feel Better* (Johns Hopkins University Press, 2013), 46.

DAY	DEPRESSED			NEUTRAL	ELEVATED MOOD			NOTES
	severe	moderate	mild	neutral	mild	moderate	severe	

TABLE 1.6. Blank Mood Chart

DAY	DEPRESSED			NEUTRAL	ELEVATED MOOD			NOTES
	severe	moderate	mild	neutral	mild	moderate	severe	
1								
2								
3								
4								
5								
6								
7								
8								
9								
10								
11								
12								
13								
14								
15								
16								
17								
18								
19								
20								
21								
22								
23								
24								
25								
26								
27								
28								
29								
30								
31								

Source: Susan J. Noonan, *Managing Your Depression: What You Can Do to Feel Better* (Johns Hopkins University Press, 2013), 46.

blood pressure, and an increased risk of diabetes and heart (cardiovascular) disease. It can lead to diabetes and long-term physical health consequences such as heart attack, stroke, kidney failure, and more. This makes it a serious medical problem, which your loved one should try to avoid if possible.

Metabolic syndrome is made up of five *cardiovascular risk factors* defined by the American Heart Association and the National Heart, Lung, and Blood Institute. A person needs to have at least three out of five of these risk factors to meet the diagnosis.

- Obesity, more prominent in the abdomen or belly (central obesity), with a waist circumference of 102 centimeters (cm) or greater in men and 88 cm or greater in women
- High triglycerides (fat) in the blood: 150 milligrams per deciliter (mg/dL) or higher
- Low HDL cholesterol in the blood (the "good" cholesterol): 40 mg/dL or less in men or 50 mg/dL or less in women
- High blood pressure: 130/85 mm Hg (millimeters of mercury) or greater, or receiving treatment for high blood pressure
- High *fasting* blood sugar: 100 mg/dL or higher (or taking medication for high blood sugar or diabetes)

Metabolic syndrome can be initially managed with lifestyle changes. These include getting adequate sleep, engaging in regular aerobic (cardiovascular) exercise and strength training, and following a low carbohydrate diet that includes healthy fats (olive oil, avocados). Sometimes medication is needed to control the elevated blood pressure, cholesterol, or blood sugar. Researchers have also looked at medications to treat the underlying inflammation associated with metabolic syndrome, but further studies are needed.

Alicia is a 42-year-old woman who has been dealing with major depression for several years. She has been on seven different antidepressant medications. Most do not help and one gave her an unpleasant side effect (headache and rash), so it had to be stopped. One course of ECT was quite effective, and now she is on a treatment combination that seems to be working well. Alicia sees a psychiatrist for management of her medications and a clinical psychologist for talk therapy, or CBT, and is making progress toward her goal of wellness.

Unfortunately, over time, Alicia has seen a 40-pound weight gain without having changed her diet or activity level. The weight is mainly in her belly. One person even thought she was pregnant! This is very upsetting to her; as is the case for many people, her image is tied into her self-esteem.

She already follows a healthy diet and exercises regularly. Alicia is quite discouraged.

Because of her unintentional weight gain, Alicia's primary care physician did some blood tests and found that she has borderline diabetes (high blood sugar), low HDL cholesterol, and slightly elevated blood pressure. She was both surprised and confused by this and spoke with a doctor at the weight center. He explained that she had metabolic syndrome *and that her depression and many of the medications used for her depression could cause it. He also said there were steps she could take to manage it, such as watching her diet and exercise routine even more closely.*

New medications to treat metabolic syndrome were discussed. She now follows a very healthy lean diet of fruits and vegetables and chicken and fish and sought a dietician's advice. He complimented her on her good food choices and recommended that she follow a Mediterranean diet. She also exercises five to six days a week, with both aerobic and strength training. She knows that sleep and stress can affect body weight and tries to manage those as well. In some people, medications are necessary to get back down to a healthy weight, and the weight center physician and she will make the best medication decision for her future health.

ANXIETY AND DEPRESSION

Anxiety along with depression is a common combination. Approximately half of those who have depression experience anxiety at the same time. In the National Comorbidity Survey (2006), 58 percent of patients aged 15 to 54 who had major depression also had an anxiety disorder. *Anxiety* is a feeling of excessive nervousness, apprehension, and worry about the future. The depth of worry, length of time it lasts, and how often it occurs is out of proportion to the actual feared event. It may cause your family member or friend to have a great deal of distress. Worry leads to a nervous and jittery feeling. He may feel restless and shaky, with trouble concentrating, irritability, and sleep difficulties. Physically, your family member could feel sweaty and shaky, as though his heart is racing or skipping a beat. An upset stomach, nausea, headache, and muscle aches are common. It all feels very real to the person at the time. Some people are frightened by these symptoms and go to the Emergency Department thinking that something is wrong with them physically.

> **Anxiety causes excessive worries that interfere with your loved one's functioning.**

Adults tend to worry about common, everyday events such as their jobs, finances, their health, the health and safety of their family members, and minor matters (doing household chores or being late for an appointment). Adolescents tend to worry excessively about their competence, appearance, fitting in socially, schoolwork, sports performance, catastrophic events (nuclear war, terrorism), or their future. In both groups, these worries are excessive, interfere with their functioning, and are of long duration and more distressing than the normal worries of everyday life.

The *DSM-5* states that in order to make a diagnosis of a generalized anxiety disorder (anxiety) a person's anxiety and worry must be associated with three or more of the following, occurring on more days than not for at least six months:

- Restlessness, or feeling keyed up or on edge
- Being easily fatigued
- Difficulty concentrating; mind going blank
- Irritability
- Muscle tension
- Sleep disturbance

The anxiety must involve a variety of events and activities such as work, school, or social performance. The individual must find it difficult to control the worry. The anxiety, worry, or physical symptoms must cause significant distress in social, occupational/school, or other areas of functioning. In addition, the disturbance must not be due to substances (drug abuse), medications, or another medical condition and is not better explained by another mental disorder.

Anxiety is a treatable condition. Medications, talk therapy, relaxation exercises, and mindfulness meditation are all effective treatment options. Lifestyle changes can reduce the symptoms, such as improving the quality and duration of sleep, getting regular physical exercise (aerobics and yoga), minimizing caffeine and alcohol use, and avoiding nicotine (tobacco) and street drugs. One key thing you can do is offer believable reassurance to your loved one. Once you are sure your family member is not having a physical medical emergency, respond with a calm, steady voice, and reassure him that he is not having a medical crisis.

Many people who experience anxiety find it helpful to do the deep breathing and relaxation exercises mentioned in chapter 9. These will often help him calm down and feel better. In addition, some new medications used to treat mood disorders can effectively treat anxiety.

STIGMA

Mood disorders such as depression and bipolar disorder still carry a stigma, even in the year 2020. A stigma arises when some misinformed people critically judge a person because of his illness and then unfairly label him with a negative stereotype or image. A person may be avoided, rejected, or shunned by others. It is a form of discrimination. Stigma can lead to an inability to make friends socially because others reject his friendship efforts, a loss of a job or earned promotion for which he is qualified, limited housing opportunities, and other unfair actions. Comments such as *You have depression—that means something's wrong with you! I can't trust you in this job*, or *You're creepy, I don't want you living next door to me* are hurtful and untrue.

> A stigma is a hurtful, negative label unfairly placed on your loved one by another person.

Some poorly informed people may believe that it is socially unacceptable to have a mood disorder. They may try to make your family member feel ashamed or disgraced because of her illness. Others may believe she is incompetent, potentially dangerous, weak in character, or undesirable just because of her illness. They will be judgmental and critical. *But they are mistaken. Their beliefs are absolutely not true.*

There is nothing unacceptable about having a biologically based condition such as depression or bipolar disorder (or diabetes or heart disease, for that matter). Unfortunately, many people are not informed about mood disorders as an illness, and they believe in the stigma, the unfair criticism, or judgment. They may try to force their inaccurate beliefs and attitudes on your loved one. Ill-informed beliefs and judgments may come from her friends, other family, or strangers who just don't know any better. These judgments may also come from the media, such as television or social media sites, which tend to sensationalize the news and perpetuate misconceptions.

> Stigma can be a barrier to your loved one's seeking professional help for mental illness, especially if she fears that others may find out and judge her negatively.

Remember that their misinformation is driving this behavior—it is not a reflection of your loved one or the reality of mood disorders.

Having an illness with a stigma attached is an additional burden for your loved one to carry on top of the depression symptoms he already feels. Having to deal with others' inaccurate reactions to and criticism of his illness can increase the suffering your loved one already experiences. He may feel he is constantly choosing whether to feel hurt and deal with that, or face the offender and correct their misinformation, if he feels he has the mental energy to do so. When others attach a stigma to your loved one's illness, it can put a strain on his relationships at home, at work, or in social situations. Remaining quiet about one's mental illness to avoid the stigma is not a good solution, however.

One effective response is for him to step back and understand that he may never be able to turn around the offending person's thinking no matter how hard he tries. Encourage him to consider the source of those distorted beliefs—and try to ignore the comments of those whose opinion he cannot change.

As a society, we have to change the mindset of those who view mood disorders negatively. Their bias is based on misinformation, fear, and arrogance. Education about depression and bipolar disorder as an illness, and the effective treatment options, is key. This will reduce the fear in people's hearts.

Signs of Depression to Look For: Making the Diagnosis

If you think your spouse, child, parent, or friend might have depression or bipolar depression, there are some things to look for that will help your efforts to assist him or her. Watch for physical changes in the person, listen to what she says and the way she says she feels, and observe the way she acts. Look for changes from her usual self in

- general appearance
- habits vital to functioning, like sleep and appetite (called *vital senses*)
- expressed feelings and attitudes about herself
- thoughts about suicide

Pay attention if you notice any of these changes in your friend or family member. Use these observations as you try to gently encourage her to seek professional help. If she's an adolescent or an elderly person under your care, it can be quite helpful to report these changes to her primary care physician or mental health providers.

GENERAL APPEARANCE

Try to think about how your family member appears in general:

Is she neat, clean, and well groomed?
Is she sloppy and disheveled or somewhere in between?
Is this different from her usual self?
Is she alert and bright or dark and moody?
Is she sad or irritable in mood, speech, or facial expression?
Does she cry frequently or snap at you?
Does she appear disinterested in her surroundings and the activities she's always liked? (For example, has she stopped participating in her weekly aerobics class or monthly book club?)
Most important, is she her usual baseline self?

Watch for your family member spending excess time alone in her room or lying on the couch watching television or staring straight ahead. One characteristic of depression is a loss of interest in life and the activities she used to enjoy. These new behaviors may indicate illness.

Ask yourself if she appears tired and fatigued or slumped over in posture or if her movements are sluggish. Note if her speech is clear or slow and muffled. Depression saps the energy out of a person, and fatigue for no other clinical reason is something significant.

Notice whether your family member is taking care of herself—attending to self-care, bathing, grooming, and wearing clean clothes. Any deviation from her typical daily habits may signal depression.

VITAL SENSES, THE HABITS VITAL TO OUR FUNCTIONING

Ask yourself if there has been any change from her usual behavior in the habits vital to daily functioning, such as sleep and appetite:

Has she gone into a pattern of sleeping more or less than usual?
Has she mentioned difficulty falling asleep, staying asleep, or waking up earlier than necessary?
Has she lost her usual amount of energy for daily life?

Note whether she takes a nap in the afternoon or early evening. Depression is often accompanied by a disruption in sleep patterns. This change could be a significant sign.

Have you seen a change in her appetite or food habits?

Does she eat more or less than usual? Eating too much, too little, skipping meals? Is it the same type of food, or has she started eating junk food or fast food? This may indicate illness as well. Has this shift in appetite or dietary habits caused a change in her body weight, such as gaining or losing five pounds or more within two weeks? In some people, depression can lead to an unintentional change in body weight over time (meaning the person did not deliberately lose or gain weight).

Do you have difficulty getting her up to go to school or work?

Does she still participate in her previous activities, including hobbies and physical exercise such as aerobics class, jogging, or basketball? Any variation in these activities, not related to a physical problem, may be a sign of depression.

Has she isolated herself from friends, family members, or prior interests and activities?

ATTITUDE ABOUT SELF

Note if her feelings and attitudes about herself and her life have changed from her usual:

> Have her thoughts about herself and her experiences become negative and distorted?
>
> Has she expressed thoughts of worthlessness or guilt?
>
> Does she have difficulty thinking, concentrating, reading, or following a conversation or television show?
>
> Has she mentioned death or suicide?
>
> Does she express inaccurate and negative thoughts about herself, such as "I'm a loser" or "Nobody ever likes me"?

Biased, automatically negative thinking can frequently occur in depression. An overview in chapter 8 describes the different types of thought distortions common to depression and may help you recognize distortions in her thinking.

Think about whether your family member has mentioned any loss of hope for her future, school, job, career, or social opportunities. Hopelessness is a key feature of this illness in many people. So is a feeling of worthlessness, in which she ignores her positive qualities, such as a sense of humor or an accomplished skill. Feeling guilty for something she had little or no control over is also worth noting.

Has she mentioned having difficulty with thinking, concentrating, reading, or following a conversation or the plot of a show on television? Trouble with concentration and focus is the top symptom of depression self-reported on the website Patients Like Me (www.patientslikeme.com).

Has she had any thoughts of death or suicide or even vaguely mentioned not wanting to "be around"? You will want to take any slight comment like this very seriously. Suicidal thoughts indicate that she requires immediate professional help.

CHECKING YOUR LOVED ONE'S BEHAVIOR

You as a family member or friend are the best one to observe your loved one's daily behavior, mood, speech, thoughts, and ability to function. You can notice any changes from his usual pattern. If any of this goes on for two weeks or longer, it is often a sign that a person is having trouble. You can be most helpful by using what you see to encourage him into mental health treatment, and/or offer that information to his providers to assist them in their decision making. Here's a checklist for you to easily capture your loved one's wayward or problematic behavior and symptoms (table 2.1). Pay attention to the actions that appear "often" in your best estimation and mention this to your loved one and her provider.

The following story about Melanie will show you how a person can have an assortment of vague symptoms noticeable to her friends and family members. The key is that, if you notice any unusual change in behavior, thoughts, or feelings in your loved one that are different from her usual self, it is advisable to encourage her to have it checked out. Many times it's the family doctor, or primary care physician, who sees the person the first time for an initial evaluation. Referral to a mental health professional may come later.

Melanie is a 28-year-old high school teacher in a suburban town. She is engaged to be married next year to her longtime boyfriend, an accountant. Her family, parents, and two sisters live about 20 minutes away. Melanie has always been considered very positive and strong, the one others lean on for support. She is even tempered, with a good sense of humor, enjoys many hobbies and sports activities, and loves shopping and dressing well, priding herself on getting a good "bargain" on her teacher's salary.

Lately, her family and fiancé have noticed some changes in Melanie. She seems to be short tempered and irritable, and many little things seem to bother her. She has no patience for others when they approach her and abruptly brushes them off. A few times she has been found crying and tearful, unusual for her, but when asked she denies any problem. Her sleep seems to be fragmented, with very early morning awakenings and some restlessness. She seems to be very tired and fatigued, just dragging around. And she appears to have lost her appetite for food, which was always quite healthy, as well as for the activities she once enjoyed like aerobics class and yoga. Melanie is usually very good at details, concentrated and focused, but lately she seems to be slipping, forgetting to do things or not remembering something.

Melanie's work attire has been noticeably more casual than usual, and her off-duty clothing is limited to leggings and sweats, which is also unusual for her. She declines going out on a shopping trip with her sister for the big sale at a local department store. She also skips washing and grooming her hair when her fiancé is not around, saying it doesn't matter. Her family is concerned by all of this, and even though she's not sad they wonder if she might be experiencing depression. They would like her primary care physician to evaluate her.

TABLE 2.1. **What I Observed**			
WHAT I OBSERVED	**ONCE-TWICE**	**OFTEN**	**WHEN IT STARTED**
Does he seem sad, depressed, or tearful?			
Is she irritable or agitated?			
Is her appearance the same as usual? Or has she stopped bathing, dressing, or caring for herself?			
Have you noticed he has lost interest or pleasure in most activities?			
Are there changes in his amount of sleep (too much or too little)?			
Is there a change in her appetite (increased or decreased) or the food she eats (junk food)?			
Has he had a weight loss or gain of 5 lb. or more in past 2 weeks without trying to?			
Does she appear fatigued, with a loss of energy?			
Have you noticed trouble in his ability to focus or concentrate on things?			
Does he seem restless; or does he appear to be physically moving very slow?			
Have you heard her talk about feeling worthless, hopeless, or guilty?			
Has he talked about death or suicide, not wanting to be here, being a burden to others?			
Have you noticed very rapid speech or racing or jumbled thoughts?			
Does she do high-risk behaviors (excessive spending, drinking, drugs, or sexual behavior)?			

MAKING THE DIAGNOSIS OF A MOOD DISORDER

There are no blood tests or X-rays for mood disorders and no high-tech scans readily available outside of a research setting. An illness of the brain leads to changes in the chemicals, cells, and structure of the brain that until recently have been difficult to observe and measure. This difficulty has meant that people have a hard time believing the disorders are real, adding to the stigma of mental illness.

Brain imaging techniques are now used in research, including magnetic resonance imaging (MRI), positron emission tomography (PET), and functional magnetic resonance imaging (fMRI). Early evidence from these scans suggests that the brains of people who have mood disorders may differ somewhat in certain places from the brains of healthy people. This is encouraging for those who have the illness, and for researchers who are working on new methods of treatment for mood disorders; it gives them some hope for developing future therapies. Note: these scans are not available at this time in clinical practice outside of a research setting, so please don't approach your provider with a request to get tested right now.

> An initial mental status exam can be done by your loved one's primary care physician or a mental health professional.

Here's what to expect when making a diagnosis of a mood disorder. In clinical practice, a thorough mental health evaluation starts with your loved one's doctor or doctors doing a number of things to make an accurate diagnosis of depression or bipolar disorder and exclude other reasons for his symptoms. Some of this may be done by his primary care physician, some by a mental health specialist. He or she will take his vital signs (heart rate, breathing rate, blood pressure, temperature, oxygen level) and do a basic physical examination.

The doctor will observe him; note his general appearance, actions, and speech (fast, slow, slurred, confused, appropriate, or inappropriate); and then ask him a detailed series of questions about how he is feeling, what kind of symptoms he is experiencing, and the kinds of thoughts he is having. Topics include sleep, appetite, weight, daily activities and interests, work or school, social supports, and thoughts of harming himself. She will test his ability to think, reason, and remember and observe his mood, thoughts, behavior, insight, judgment, and affect (how he expresses emotion), for example, does he laugh or cry? This is the *mental health assessment* or *mental status exam*. Oftentimes, you will be invited into the examination room, with your loved one's permission, and asked questions about what you've observed.

Your loved one will also be asked about his family's medical history—what illnesses "run" in your family—to see whether anything else may account for his symptoms. Next, blood and urine tests will be done to make sure that no other physical problem is causing the illness, such as a thyroid condition, illicit drugs in his system such as cocaine or methamphetamine (these would appear on a toxicology blood test), or other prescribed medications such as steroids (prednisone) or others (see table 14.1).

After pulling all of this information together, the doctor will conclude with a diagnosis and either start treatment or refer your family member to a mental health specialist for consultation and more specific therapy.

Healthy Ways to Handle Mood Disorders

What happens when your loved one first suspects that he or she has a mood disorder such as major depression or bipolar disorder or has been diagnosed by a qualified mental health professional? The best results or outcomes are found in those who learn about the illness and how to manage it and who master the following steps. The goal is to prevent recurrence (a return of symptoms) of major depression or mania, to reduce the burden of symptoms, and to improve functioning in between mood episodes. How does your loved one do this?

Educating oneself about mood disorders can be done with the help of an individual therapist, in family or couples' therapy, or in a psychoeducational support group, presentation or seminar. When your loved one makes the effort to educate himself about his mood disorder and the management of it, the effect will be fewer symptoms of depression or mania, a greater chance of sticking with recommended medications and treatments, a longer time in between episodes (increased time to recurrence) with fewer recurrences over time, and fewer or no inpatient hospital admissions. He will feel better overall. It's hard work and not easy to do at first and will take a lot of patience and persistence on his part, with a lot of support from you. The steps follow:

- *Illness awareness.* Your loved one will have to come to terms with having a mood disorder and accepting the diagnosis. She will need to become aware that her feelings are symptoms of an illness and are not facts. With major depression, she will have to accept that the illness has episodes that come and go over time in an unpredictable pattern unique to her. With bipolar disorder, a person will have to accept that this chronic, or lifelong, illness requires daily medications to remain stable. She will need to become aware of the symptoms, warning signs, and personal triggers that may signal the course of her depression or mania. All mood disorders will require an adjustment in lifestyle to some extent and perhaps in her life goals and daily activities. Many times a person has a lack of insight into their illness, which presents an additional obstacle to acceptance. If your loved one denies having a mood disorder and refuses to follow a treatment plan, that will only extend her emotional pain and misery. You will need to be firm yet patient as she moves through this process of acceptance.

- *Sticking to treatment.* Taking a medication, attending a weekly support group, or following health-promoting behaviors (getting enough sleep, eating well, exercising) are not too hard to do for a week or two for most of us. The challenge is committing to these activities for a lifetime, accepting that fact and the necessity, and keeping yourself motivated. Psychiatric medications and treatments characteristically take several weeks before you see the effects, sometimes up to six to eight weeks, and in that time it's very difficult to stick with the treatment regimen when your loved one feels that he isn't seeing any positive results yet. In a sense, he's following a course of treatment on blind faith, based on the confidence and trust he has in his mental health clinician. This is where it is important to find a provider with a "good fit" and an effective treatment alliance. The person who has the mood disorder is often the last one to see any signs of improvement. It's usually noticed first by friends and family members, and he may often deny it! You may observe a slight lift in his mood, less irritability, a smile or a laugh on occasion, things like that. Take the opportunity to point these out to your loved one so that he has markers of his progress and a way to keep motivated.

- *Detection of early warning signs.* Each person who has a mood disorder has a characteristic set of signs that signal a change is going on in his or her illness. These are *warning signs*, which you may observe as distinct changes from his baseline that precede a depressive or manic episode. It might be changes in your loved one's thoughts, behaviors, daily routine, or self-care activities. You might notice that your loved one feels less hopeful, is more irritable, has a change in his sleep pattern, has difficulty with daily household or work routines, or has stopped bathing as often. Early recognition of these unique warning signs gives your loved one and his treatment team a chance to intervene and modify (change or improve) the course of his illness. Intervention might include an adjustment in dose, frequency, or type of medication or a different tactic in talk therapy.

- *Lifestyle patterns.* Those who have a mood disorder are greatly helped by keeping up a regular pattern of healthy lifestyle habits. This includes taking medications as prescribed, following a regular sleep schedule seven days per week, eating healthy food three meals a day, having daily physical exercise, keeping a structure and routine to your day, and avoiding isolation by keeping up with friends and family members. Once this becomes habit, a person actually feels better, has greater energy, and doesn't have to put forth effort into thinking about it. These are discussed in detail in the next section.

THE BASICS OF MENTAL HEALTH

Just like the rest of our body, our brain needs continuous care to function well. The most effective way to have a healthy brain is to try to follow a set of daily self-help steps called the Basics of Mental Health (Noonan 2013) that I learned about in reading many sources about depression and as a patient at McLean Hospital in Belmont, Massachusetts. These essentials for maintaining emotional health and stability include a regular pattern of sleep, diet, and exercise, as well as taking medications as advised, having a daily routine and structure, and having frequent contact with nontoxic friends and family. The Basics are part of our normal lives and are not exotic or unusual in any way, but sometimes, especially when fatigued, we forget to pay attention to them. Building these steps into your daily routine means they become habit, and you don't have to think much about doing them, which is the goal.

Your family member or friend may find any one or all of these challenging to do while depressed and dealing with the symptoms of a mood disorder. That's because the symptoms of depression or bipolar disorder often interfere with one's ability to follow these Basics. For example, with depression it becomes more difficult to find the energy to exercise, to shop for healthy groceries and eat well, or to pick up the phone and interact with friends. Yet these are the steps that help to improve the symptoms of depression, and sound scientific information supports this. It takes hard work and perseverance to follow the basics when depressed, but when it gets your loved one out of a deep hole, he'll see that the results are worth it.

You as a friend or family member can take on the role of coach and gently encourage him to stick to these Basics, one at a time. You may also choose to adopt a few of these healthy guidelines for yourself. By doing so, you become an example of a healthy lifestyle and role model for your family member or friend. Doing the Basics together may make it easier for him to follow them. This means that you try to keep regular sleep hours yourself, prepare nutritious meals for the family, and don't stock junk foods in the kitchen. You might offer to join your family member or friend for a walk or bike ride outdoors, encourage him to connect with other friends and family, and help him keep to a routine and daily structure by getting him an agenda book to plan and write down even the smallest daily activities.

The Basics of Mental Health are listed in more detail:

- Treat any physical illness
- Sleep
  - Aim for seven to eight hours of sleep each night.
  - Go to bed and wake up at the same time every day of the week, including nonwork and nonschool days. Keep a regular sleep routine.
  - Keep your sleep environment quiet and relaxing.
  - Reserve the bed for sleep and sex only and no other activities such as eating, working, reading, watching television, and so on.
  - Track your sleep routine with a sleep diary and share it with your doctor.
  - Follow the sleep hygiene guidelines to promote restful sleep (table 3.1).
- Diet and nutrition
  - Eat three healthy, balanced meals each day.
  - Avoid street drugs and alcohol.
  - Limit caffeine intake.
  - For basic nutritional guidelines, see www.choosemyplate.gov and USDA *Dietary Guidelines for Americans 2015–2020* (table 3.2).
- Medications
  - Take all medications as prescribed.
  - Talk to your doctor about the use of vitamins and herbal supplements.
- Exercise regularly
  - Seek a balance of cardiovascular, strength training, and stretch and relaxation activities three to five days per week.
  - Strive for 150 to 300 minutes of moderate exercise per week or 75 minutes of vigorous exercise per week (*Physical Activity Guidelines for Americans*, US Department of Health and Human Services [HHS] 2018).

- Maintain positive social contact with your friends and family on a regular basis. Avoid isolation.
- Have a routine and structure to each day
  - Structure your time each day (doesn't have to be rigid!).
  - Write your daily tasks and appointments in an electronic or paper agenda.
  - Break large tasks into small steps.
  - Include positive, pleasurable experiences in your day as well as home, family, and work responsibilities.

Sleep

You might wonder how and why these Basics have an impact on your family member's or friend's mood and depression symptoms. Sleep is essential for all of us to function well. We need sleep for our bodies and brains to restore and repair the effects of the day. People often find that sleep problems occur during an episode of depression or bipolar disorder. Your family member or friend may sleep too much, too little, or in fragmented bursts. If manic, she may be energized and require little sleep. Normally, healthy adults require, on average, seven to nine hours per night of uninterrupted sleep, but after age 60, nighttime sleep tends to be shorter, lighter, and interrupted by multiple awakenings.

> Sound sleep optimizes brain function and is thought to have a positive effect on mood.

Without enough sleep, your family member may become irritable, experience fatigue, or have trouble concentrating. A change in sleep can also affect depression and bipolar disorder and might trigger an episode. Cognitive Behavior Therapy for Insomnia (CBT-I), which is done with a clinical psychologist or a therapist, is the first-line treatment for those who have sleep problems. It addresses the thoughts, beliefs, and behaviors about sleep that contribute to persistent sleep problems.

To optimize her sleep, your loved one can attend to the principles of sleep hygiene. *Sleep hygiene* refers to the personal habits and environmental conditions (what it's like in her bedroom) that affect a person's sleep, including *not* eating, reading, working, or watching TV in bed; instead, the bed should be reserved for sleep or sex. Avoid being stimulated at bedtime (by invigorating music, TV, conversations or phone calls, or blue light from electronic devices). Exposure to blue wavelength light from electronic devices and your smartphone, tablet, computer, fluorescent or LED light bulbs, and TV at night interferes with the body's production and secretion of melatonin, a hormone involved in regulating our normal sleep-wake cycles.

Paying attention to sleep hygiene helps to reduce the behaviors and habits that can interfere with sleep or stimulate us around bedtime. It's important for everyone, but especially those who have mood disorders, to keep good sleep habits and a consistent sleeping pattern in a bedroom that favors sound sleep. It's something that your loved one has control over. Essential elements to put into place that will help your loved one get a restful night's sleep are listed in table 3.1. If this does not work, it's time to speak with the family physician.

Feed your body. Feed your brain.

Nutrition

The next essential on the list of Basics is nutrition. Food is the fuel that keeps our brains and bodies operating properly, and the quality of that food affects the health of our hearts, lungs, and brain. If a person skips meals or relies on unhealthy choices, junk food, or illicit drugs, the brain does not function well, leading to physical and mental fatigue and irritability. A poor or irregular diet, or one of highly processed foods, may make your family member or friend vulnerable to depression. A balanced whole food diet high in nutrient dense foods comprised of whole fruits, a variety of colorful vegetables, whole grains, beans, fish, poultry, and a small amount of olive oil improves mood and is associated with a lower rate of depression. A healthy diet improves the kinds of bacteria that normally live inside our gut or intestines (called the gut microbiome), which promotes brain health and a normal body weight. The Mediterranean diet is often recommended as a healthy option and is easy to follow. Dr. Felice Jacka, a Professor of Nutrition and Epidemiologic Psychiatry at Deakin University in Australia, is considered a world leader on this subject and has written a book called *Brain Changer: The Good Mental Health Diet* (2019), which may be of interest to you.

Eat real food. Avoid processed food.

For help with healthy meal preparation, the United States Department of Agriculture (USDA) has an easy-to-follow interactive website at www.choosemyplate.gov with information about balanced meals and healthy portion sizes. For most of us, the visual image displayed on this site is a meaningful and memorable way to keep our meals on track, since it's much easier to remember these simple pictures. In addition, the HHS and the USDA jointly publish online dietary guidelines for healthy eating (www.dietaryguidelines.gov). These are included in table 3.2, which is a summary of the key points from the USDA dietary guidelines.

These *Dietary Guidelines for Americans 2015–2020* display healthy food as portions divided on a dinner plate with fruits, vegetables, whole grains, lean

TABLE 3.1. **Sleep Hygiene**

Recommendations to improve your sleep include:

- Keep the same bedtime and wake-up time every day, including weekends. Set an alarm clock if necessary. Get up and out of bed at the same time every morning, even if you've had a bad night's sleep.

- Avoid napping during the day.

- Develop a relaxing ritual before bedtime. Create "downtime" during the last 2 hours before sleep and avoid overstimulation.

- Try going to bed only when you are sleepy.

- Avoid watching the clock or lying in bed frustrated at being unable to fall asleep. Turn the clock away from you.

- If you're unable to fall asleep after 20 to 30 minutes, get out of bed. Relax and distract your mind with a quiet activity in another room (music, reading). Return to bed when you feel sleepy.

- Relaxation exercises before bedtime may help. Examples include progressive muscle relaxation, deep breathing, guided imagery, yoga, or meditation.

- Designate a specific "worry time" earlier in the day or evening to sort out any problems. Writing down reminders for the next day helps to clear your mind before bed.

- Use your bed and bedroom only for sleep, sex, or occasional illness. Eliminate non-sleep activities in bed. Use another room for reading, television, work, or eating.

- Limit the use of caffeine during the day and avoid its use after 12:00 p.m. Note that coffee, tea, colas, chocolate, and some medications contain caffeine.

- Avoid or limit the use of nicotine (tobacco) and alcohol during the day. Don't use them within 4 to 6 hours of bedtime.

- Avoid large meals before bedtime, but don't go to bed hungry. If needed, have a light snack.

- Exercise on a regular basis. Avoid strenuous exercise within 4 to 6 hours of bedtime.

- Create a bedroom environment that favors sound sleep. A comfortable bed in a dark, quiet room is recommended. Minimize light, noise, and hot or cold extremes in room temperature. Room-darkening shades, curtains, earplugs, or a sound machine may be helpful.

- Speak with your doctor if you are having continued difficulty with sleep, including falling asleep, staying asleep, and early or frequent awakenings.

Source: Susan J. Noonan, *Managing Your Depression: What You Can Do to Feel Better* (Johns Hopkins University Press, 2013), 8–9. *Additional References:* American Academy of Sleep Medicine, Healthy Sleep Habits, http://sleepeducation.org/essentials-in-sleep/healthy-sleep-habits, accessed March 2019; National Sleep Foundation, Sleep Hygiene, https://www.sleepfoundation.org/articles/sleep-hygiene, accessed March 2019.

protein, and a small amount of low-fat dairy. Portion control is important, as we've become used to an increased portion size of entrées, muffins, sodas—nearly everything—in our society over the past 10 to 20 years. The guidelines recommend that half of your plate consist of fruits and vegetables or that you eat five one-half-cup servings of colorful fruits and vegetables each day. For adults, the protein portion should be five to six ounces total of lean meat, poultry, fish, or eggs each day (divided among your meals). Grains

---

TABLE 3.2. USDA Dietary Guidelines for Americans 2015–2020

Here's a summary list of the key points important to maintaining a healthy body and weight.

- Include a large amount of whole grains, colorful vegetables, and fruits in your diet.

- Eat a variety of vegetables, especially dark green, red, and orange vegetables and beans and peas.

- Replace refined grains with whole grains. At least half of all grains eaten should be whole grains.

- Choose a variety of protein foods, which include seafood, lean meat and poultry, eggs, beans and peas, soy products, and unsalted nuts and seeds. Choose seafood in place of some meat and poultry.

- Use lean, lower calorie proteins instead of high-fat protein.

- Reduce your amount of sugar-sweetened beverages.

- Focus on the total number of calories consumed. Monitor your food intake.

- Be aware of portion size: choose smaller portions or lower-calorie options.

- Eat a nutrient-dense breakfast.

- Reduce daily sodium (salt) intake to less than 2,300 milligrams (mg) per day.

- Get less than 10% of calories from saturated fatty acids. Replace them with monounsaturated and polyunsaturated fatty acids.

- Eat fewer than 300 mg per day of dietary cholesterol.

- Increase fat-free or low-fat milk and milk products, such as milk, yogurt, cheese, or fortified soy beverages.

- Use oils to replace solid fats when possible.

- Choose foods that are a rich source of potassium, dietary fiber, calcium, and vitamin D. These include vegetables, fruits, whole grains, and milk and milk products.

- Limit foods that contain synthetic sources of trans fats, such as partially hydrogenated oils.

Source: USDA Dietary Guidelines for Americans, 2015–2020, 8th ed., December 2015.

should ideally be three ounces of whole grains per serving. Dairy should be low fat and used in moderation, as should oil. Trans fats should be avoided completely.

Emily, in this next story, shows us how a mood disorder, such as major depression or bipolar disorder, can affect a person's ability to care for herself in healthy ways, such as with a good diet and regular physical exercise. The affected person is often just too tired and disinterested to do these things. This vignette illustrates creative ways that family members and friends can help their loved one deal with basic needs and may be something you'd like to try. You may have already thought of other methods.

Emily is a 32-year-old single woman who lives alone in a studio apartment. She has a good job as an administrative assistant. Her parents and younger brother live in a suburb about 30 minutes away; she speaks with them regularly and sees them occasionally on weekends and holidays. For the past two years, she has been treated for major depressive disorder and has recently become quite discouraged. She is overwhelmed by fatigue and lack of energy to do even the simple things each day, such as laundry, grocery shopping, and cooking for herself. Sometimes Emily relies on takeout, frozen entrées, or cereal and bananas for dinner, or she skips meals entirely. She stopped exercising and going to the gym because it was just too much to do. Because of this, she has gained ten pounds and feels bad about herself and her self-image and has lost interest in dating. Her mother has tried to help but doesn't know what to do.

Recently, her cousin Clara moved nearby, and she had a few ideas to help Emily. First, Clara came over and together they went out on a fifteen-minute brisk walk around the block on two evenings after work and on Saturday mornings. Emily was surprised to discover that, in fact, she could do it and that she felt a bit better. Next, Clara planned that together they would go food shopping on Sunday mornings, before the crowds got there, to stock up on healthy foods for the whole week. Clara also had Emily prepare a list of shopping items in advance to make their trip more efficient. That went pretty well.

Then Clara said, "We're going to have a cooking fest! Every other Sunday afternoon, I will come to your apartment, we'll put on some good rockin' music, and cook up a few different healthy foods in batches and freeze them in individual portions for you to have for the next week." They made things like chicken and broccoli, beans and rice, soups, and stew. At first, Clara brought over easy recipes with five ingredients or fewer that she found online. When this plan was going well, she asked Emily to search out her own simple healthy recipes; things she might like to try. This was a success! Emily now had good food options that she could defrost quickly or perhaps add fresh vegetables or a salad to them. It was also much less expensive than takeout. She began to feel better, more energized. Their walks became more vigorous and extended to thirty minutes at a time, and she started to lose some weight. Her fatigue and self-esteem began to improve, as did her depression.

Exercise

The next Basic, regular physical exercise, is equally good for our brain and its ability to function optimally. Moderate-to-vigorous physical activity improves mood, enriches the quality of sleep, and promotes improvements in executive functioning, which is the ability to plan and organize, self-monitor, initiate tasks, and control our emotions. Physical exercise decreases the risk of clinical depression and anxiety; it also improves our quality of life and physical functioning. And the opposite is true. The lack of exercise—being sedentary or sitting for three or more hours per day—is related to higher rates of depression. In a recent study (Choi 2019) using genetics to look at the impact of exercise on mood, researchers found that engaging in physical activity is associated with a reduced risk for depression and may be an effective preventive strategy.

> **Exercise can both improve depression symptoms and prevent symptoms.**

In several combined reviews of depression research studies (called meta-analyses), exercise was associated with an improvement in the rating scores of depression (where a lower score is better) compared with a "no exercise" group. Exercise appears to have both a therapeutic and preventive effect on the course of depression; it can both make it better and prevent it from occurring in the first place. In another research study (Harvey 2018) where the scientists followed a group of 33,908 persons for 11 years, they found that regular physical exercise (at least one hour each week) was associated with fewer episodes of future depression but not anxiety. In addition, exercise may also counteract the sense of fatigue that comes along with depression.

Physical exercise can affect our brains in a few good ways. Scientists have recently learned that when a person exercises the body releases certain chemicals (proteins) in the brain in addition to the feel-good *endorphins* you may have heard about. These chemicals, or *brain derived neurotrophic factor* (BDNF), act like fertilizer for the brain and promote the growth of new brain cells and the growth of new connections between brain cells. This process is boosted by mental exercises, aerobic physical exercise, good nutrition, and sleep and by keeping socially active. It's a possibility that was unheard of ten years ago. So, it's one way for your family member or friend to help herself that she has control over, a way to take a more active role in managing her depression.

Physical exercise has many benefits: in our body and mind and as a treatment for depression, but we often don't think of it in that way. The benefits of exercise are that it

- increases a brain chemical called BDNF, which promotes the growth of new brain cells and the connections between brain cells
- helps to regulate certain brain chemicals (neurotransmitters)
- helps to keep the level of stress hormones normal, relieving stress
- increases feelings of confidence, self-esteem, competence, and mastery
- has a positive effect on a person's mood
- improves his sense of well-being
- releases the feel-good hormones (endorphins)
- improves the quality of sleep, which in turn improves his mood disorder
- helps to overcome the inertia and sedentary lifestyle that often comes with depression;
- increases your loved one's social contacts (such as when he participates in an exercise class or in neighborhood or health club interactions)
- builds endurance and physical strength, which combats fatigue
- helps manage body weight

Regular exercise may be helpful alone or when combined with standard antidepressant treatment. This is called an *augmentation strategy*. Before beginning an exercise program, your family member should discuss his plan with his primary care physician. Have him mention any physical health concerns, such as heart disease or bone or joint problems.

What does exercise consist of? Exercise is any repeated physical activity or movement of the body that is planned, structured, and repetitive intended to improve and maintain health and physical fitness. During exercise, a person generally gets sweaty, breathes heavy, and increases his heart rate. The American College of Sports Medicine considers that a regular physical exercise program is essential for most adults. It's recommended that we all do a combination of

- aerobic activities that increase our heart rate and breathing (see the examples in table 3.3);
- strength activities, which means moving in a controlled way against a force or resistance that builds and maintains bones and muscle; and
- balance and stretching activities that increase physical stability and flexibility, such as yoga, tai chi, or basic stretches.

It's smart that we all pay more attention to our activity level. A survey of the US population looked at trends in sedentary behavior (inactivity) from 2001 to 2016 and found the frequency of sitting to watch television or videos for at least two hours per day was high in all age groups, ranging from 62 percent in children to 84 percent in senior adults. Likewise, the frequency of computer use outside of school or work increased among all age groups, and the estimated time spent sitting increased among adolescents and adults. Sedentary behavior, which means sitting without physical activity, is associated with many preventable health issues, such as heart disease, diabetes, cancer, obesity, and other chronic illnesses.

The United States Department of Health and Human Services in collaboration with the Centers for Disease Control and Prevention, the National Institutes of Health, and the President's Council on Sports, Fitness and Nutrition have put together a set of physical activity guidelines for Americans for all age groups. The physical activity guidelines recommend that adults get

- at least 150 to 300 minutes of moderate intensity physical activity per week *and* muscle strength training on two or more days of the week or
- at least 75 minutes of vigorous intensity physical activity per week *and* strength training on two or more days of the week.
- flexibility and balance exercises at least twice per week.

These guidelines include separate activity sections with specifications for children, older adults over age 65, physical activity during pregnancy and postpartum and for adults who have a chronic health condition.

When a person does aerobic exercise, his body's large muscles (such as the quadriceps or hamstring muscles in the legs) move for a sustained period, his heart rate and breathing rate increase, and he gets sweaty. A workout might be a brisk walk, run, bicycle ride, swim, or session on an elliptical trainer. There are three parts to aerobic exercise that influence the amount of benefit one gets from each workout: intensity, frequency, and duration. *Intensity* is how hard you work, *frequency* is how often you do the activity, and *duration* is how long. For example, your loved one might work out for 30 minutes per session (duration) three times per week (frequency) with moderate effort (intensity). Examples of exercise intensity are found in table 3.3.

Strength activities are those that cause the body's muscles to work against a force or resistance, as when your loved one picks up something heavy like a weight or presses against a resistance band. Building muscle keeps our body strong and helps burn more calories. This is because muscle burns more calories than does fat or bone and adding muscle by strength training increases the energy one uses daily. We also burn more calories for 72 hours after a strength-training workout.

Muscle-strengthening activities also have three components that influence the amount of benefit one gets from the exercise: intensity, repetitions, and frequency. A person might lift 20 pounds of weight (intensity) 15 times (repetitions) three days per week (frequency).

TABLE 3.3 **Examples of Exercise Intensity**	
MODERATE INTENSITY ACTIVITY	**VIGOROUS INTENSITY ACTIVITY**
• Walking (2.5–3.5 mph)	• Walking fast (4–4.5 mph)
• Water aerobics	• Jogging or running (5.0 mph or faster)
• Biking on level ground	• Swimming laps
• Playing tennis—doubles	• Taking an aerobics or spinning class
• Mowing the lawn	• Using aerobic equipment (elliptical trainer, etc.)
• Cleaning the house	• Biking fast or up hills
• Dancing	• Playing tennis—singles
• Canoeing, kayaking	• Playing basketball
• Golfing	• Playing soccer
• Gardening	• Heavy gardening
• Playing baseball or softball	• Hiking uphill
• Playing with children	• Jumping rope

Source: Adapted from US Department of Health and Human Services, *Physical Activity Guidelines for Americans*, HHS, 2018, Table 4.1, https://health.gov/paguidelines/second-edition/pdf/Physical_Activity_Guidelines_2nd_edition.pdf#page=55.

Resistance training decreases the belly fat commonly seen in older men and women and in metabolic syndrome; increases our physical functioning; decreases the chance of getting type 2 diabetes; decreases resting blood pressure; increases bone density; decreases fatigue, anxiety, and depression; and improves cognitive abilities and self-esteem.

Move more. Sit less.

To balance out our physical activities, *stretch and flexibility, balance, relaxation,* and perhaps a *meditation* routine have also been found to be helpful. It's good for the body physically and mentally and keeps the level of stress hormones normal, relieving stress and benefiting your loved one's mood in a positive way. Stretch activities, and those that improve our balance, such as yoga, tai chi, or progressive muscle relaxation for each major muscle group, also increase physical stability and flexibility. Several times per week, encourage your family member to take a few minutes to sit and relax each muscle in his body from head to toe, one muscle at a time, for about 20 seconds each, starting with the jaw, neck, shoulders, arms, and fingers. Doing this after physical exercise is often a good moment to try it.

Other relaxation techniques that many people have found helpful are visualization (sit and focus on a serene, calm image or favorite place for 5 to 10 minutes at a time, several times per week), deep-breathing exercises, and meditation. *The Relaxation Response* (Benson 2000) describes how to get started. For more information on relaxation and coping techniques, see my book for people who have a mood disorder, *Take Control of Your Depression: Strategies to Help You Feel Better Now* (2018).

How to begin. A physical exercise program is hard to do when your family member is dealing with depression. The fatigue and lack of interest and motivation common in depression often get in the way of starting and keeping up an exercise routine. Depression symptoms may also make it more difficult to exercise, including loss of interest in activities, decreased physical and mental energy, decreased motivation, and loss of focus and concentration.

To begin, first, help your family member choose an exercise activity that he enjoys—or used to enjoy—knows how to do and can realistically do on a regular basis. This is not really the time to learn something brand new and complicated. Once he picks his preferred exercise program, sticking with it is the most important part. *So how does he do that when depressed?* That's a major challenge! One trick is to make exercise part of his daily routine and schedule it as a key part of his day. Here is where *action precedes motivation.* This means that your loved one would start his exercise program now and keep at it, even if he doesn't really feel like doing it. The motivation for doing it will come later (table 3.4).

TABLE 3.4. Get Started with Exercise and Keep It Going!

- Do what you enjoy or used to enjoy. Do something fun.

- Assess what type of exercise resources are available to you. Look for a safe area to walk in your neighborhood. Find out if there is a community center or health club facility available to you with exercise classes or equipment. Consider whether you have or can invest in home exercise equipment. See what kind of social supports are available to keep you motivated to exercise.

- Plan a specific and realistic activity that you can do. Define the type of activity, how often you will do it, and for how long (frequency and duration).

- Make exercise a priority in your day and a key part of your daily routine.

- Believe that the exercise will benefit you—this will make it easier to do.

- List the pros and cons of exercising compared to having a sedentary lifestyle.

- Come up with your own personal reasons for exercising.

- Exercise with a partner (a walking partner or people in a class)— you will have to be accountable to him or her to show up and exercise together. This is a good social support.

- Consider having a personal trainer help you set up a program and then monitor and motivate you.

- Identify and address any barriers ahead of time, such as the time of day, your energy level, balancing other obligations, too busy, too tired, too sick, bored, embarrassed, and so forth.

- Work toward a goal that has personal meaning. This could be a walking or running distance, or length of time or a specific exercise accomplishment.

- Train for a charity event (such as a walk-, run-, or bike-a-thon).

- Track your progress in a journal or log and review it periodically.

- Focus on the activity and not on your performance. Try not to make comparisons to your past or others' performance.

- As you get stronger, vary your activity so that you avoid boredom and repetitive injury.

- Give yourself credit for what you can do now.

If he or she hasn't exercised in a while, it's recommended that he start slowly and gradually build up his time and effort. He might commit to walking around the block for 10 minutes three days per week and then gradually increase the amount of time each day and the number of days per week. He should set realistic, achievable goals and incorporate small changes into his daily activities, such as walking more places, taking the stairs instead of the elevator, or getting off the subway or bus two stops early.

Some find it helpful to have an "exercise buddy" or partner who will help to motivate or encourage them. It's harder to back out or make excuses when someone is waiting for you to show up. This is where you as a support person can come in and be the exercise partner for your loved one. Commit to a time, a place, and a type of activity that you will do together and hold him to it.

Tracking her progress is also a very good way for your family member to monitor her activities, to adjust her exercise routine as she gets stronger, and to help to keep up her motivation. Record the type and duration of physical activities in a weekly agenda or exercise log. There are also many electronic gadgets for this purpose, such as a Fitbit or smartphone downloadable exercise apps. As your loved one keeps up with her exercise program, her strength, endurance, and energy level will improve. The more she does, the stronger she will become, and the more likely she will do the activity. The best advice I have read is for the person to get fit and continue to challenge herself, raising the bar periodically. The more fit she is physically, the more resilient her brain will become and the better it will function.

Avoid Isolation

The next Basic of mental health concerns those who have depression and tend to isolate themselves, withdrawing from their usual activities and their friends and family. Your family member or friend may prefer to stay at home, stop answering the phone, and stay in her sweats all day. It's a huge effort to get out and interact with people when depressed. Social isolation can have a big impact on mood, however, driving it down even more. Encourage your loved one to get out, see people, and do some of the things she used to enjoy, even if she doesn't find pleasure in them right now. I personally follow the mantra *action precedes motivation*. This means that you try to get her started on something, anything, which is hard to do when she does not feel like doing it. The interest and motivation for doing it will follow later. Keeping up with social contacts may help maintain emotional well-being and protect against depression.

Structure and Routine

A routine and structure to one's day can counteract the overwhelming impact of some symptoms like lethargy, fatigue, and loss of interest in activities. It gives a person an overall sense of purpose, a feeling of accomplishment, and control of his life. Your family member or friend should try to have a routine and schedule his day without being too rigid. He may find it easy to use a paper or an electronic agenda that he can carry around and refer to frequently. He could include in it his work and home responsibilities, daily self-care, physical exercise schedule, social contacts, and positive experiences (see examples in table 3.5). It's most useful if he keeps it prioritized, with a time frame and specific, attainable, and realistic items. Sticky notes are also useful as reminders.

> Empty hours of unscheduled or alone time frequently worsen the symptoms of depression.

In this next story, we can see how depression often interferes with a person's ability to get things done, the little things in life that might feel overwhelming to do. It shows the benefits of having a simple system in place to keep tract of our daily tasks. We don't all know how to do this automatically, and some of us are naturally more organized than others, and that's when it's time to call for some help. Putting a system in place, any system, is bound to decrease stress and anxiety, minimize family tensions, and give us a sense of accomplishment. It will also help us avoid the hassles of forgotten unpaid bills, neglected household duties, and strained relationships.

Karen is a 67-year-old married mother of three who has been a homemaker for the past 38 years. Her children are grown, and her grandchildren are in high school and no longer need her on a regular basis. Her husband is often busy at work or playing golf on weekends. Karen has been treated for bipolar depression for many years, and it has been stable, yet she feels that she cannot get a handle on her life. She can't seem to remember all the little things she needs to do for herself, her children, and their household, and lately she doesn't seem to care if she forgets. She can't seem to focus and concentrate on the complexities of maintaining a household, helping out her children and grandchildren, or addressing her own needs. Sometimes the laundry or grocery shopping doesn't get done, or she doesn't shower, because she's too overwhelmed or fatigued by her depression, and that's been difficult to explain to her family. Sometimes she would just sit and stare into space for hours at a time. Last week Karen forgot about her grandson's dentist appointment, made months ago. Papers pile up on the kitchen counter, phone calls to the plumber don't seem to get made, and some things never get done despite her goal to maintain a smooth household and family. This makes her husband angry, and they argue over this. And it's discouraging to Karen, because she is much more organized when she is well.

Karen spoke with her therapist about this, and together they found a peer support person, someone who was also trained in organizational skills, to work with her. The peer understood her dilemma and her illness and came up with several suggestions. First was to have a working calendar or agenda with the days of the week spread out to be seen at a glance. It was Karen's choice as to whether this would be electronic computer-based or paper; either would work well. Karen's job was to fill it in, add the essential items, even seemingly small ones like "do laundry" or "meet Jenny for coffee." Next was to create a to-do list for each day and week and prioritize what would go on that list in small, achievable, and realistic steps. She could even color code it using sticky notes, with a different color signifying each priority or child and revise as needed. There is some satisfaction and sense of accomplishment in checking off completed items. Karen started with these few organizational ideas, stuck with them on most days, and over time noticed a greater sense of control in her life and her illness.

TABLE 3.5. Pleasurable Activities

Relax (on your own or use a relaxation CD)

Stretch

Get physical exercise

Go for a walk outdoors

Enjoy the weather

Bicycle

Garden

Play a sport

Watch sports

Play a game

Spend time with friends

Read the comics

Plan a party

Go to a party

Give someone a gift

Watch a good or funny movie

Laugh

Shop or window shop

Knit, crochet, or needlepoint

Do woodworking projects

Enjoy a good fragrance or smell

Pamper yourself (bubble bath, etc.)

Get a massage

Have your hair done

Get a manicure or pedicure

Visit a museum

Cook

Eat a good meal

Go on a date

Enjoy quiet time

Meditate

Work on a favorite project

Learn something new

Reach a goal

Travel

Work on a favorite hobby

Read a good book or magazine

Spend time with family you enjoy

Spend time with children

Volunteer

Do a jigsaw puzzle

Do Sudoku

Do a crossword puzzle

Play with a pet

Listen to music

Attend a concert

Play an instrument

Sing

Learn a new language

Look at beautiful scenery

Gaze at beautiful art

And lots of other things . . .

4

Finding Professional Help

PROFESSIONAL HELP

Although you are doing the best you can, at some point you may find that your family member needs the assistance of a mental health professional. This can be a big decision for you and your family. Where to begin? You have so many things to consider and so many choices. You may wonder when the time is right to set this up. Sometimes, it's difficult to know. The key is that any persistent change in your family member's usual self signals that a professional evaluation would be helpful.

You are often the *first* one to notice changes in your loved one's mental health.

Most often it is you, the family members and close friends, who recognize the first signs of depression in your loved one. Family members are often the ones who encourage someone's self-care and early treatment. You may notice small changes well before a physician or therapist who does not know him as you do. Your loved one most likely respects your opinion and observations and will listen to your recommendations. This may help him take the necessary steps to obtain professional help.

Mental Health Providers

Many people in your position find it overwhelming to decide among the different types of outpatient mental health professionals. How do you help your family member pick a provider? What do their different credentials mean? To begin, choosing a mental health provider depends on your family member's needs. As you will learn when you read on, there are different types of providers, each with different training and skills. Selecting the category of professional is the first step. The next decision depends in part on who is practicing in his local area; their availability; and to a certain extent, your family member's insurance coverage (for example, which providers are in his insurance plan's network and therefore more affordable).

Your family member can also start with his primary care physician (PCP) or family doctor, who will ask him questions about how he is feeling and doing, assess his situation, evaluate his depression briefly, and either begin treatment right away or refer him to a specialist in treating people who have mental health problems. It may take a while to diagnose the depression and to find a mental health provider with whom he feels comfortable. Some PCPs are experienced in treating early depression, and that may be just what he needs. But more severe types of depression may require a mental health specialist.

You will discover several different types of mental health professionals who are qualified to treat depression. They often work together as a team (table 4.1):

TABLE 4.1. **Who's Who in an Outpatient Depression Treatment Team**	
PSYCHIATRISTS	Medical doctors who are specialty trained, licensed, and board certified in psychiatry to treat mental illnesses such as depression, bipolar disorder, anxiety, and other conditions. They can evaluate individuals for a disorder and prescribe medications such as antidepressants.
PSYCHOLOGISTS	Mental health clinical specialists who have obtained their master's degree or PhD in clinical psychology and who are trained and licensed to evaluate and treat using various kinds of talk therapy. Psychologists are sometimes referred to as therapists.
SOCIAL WORKERS	Licensed clinical social workers (LICSW or LCSW) are trained to provide talk therapy to individuals or groups of people.
NURSE PRACTITIONERS	Some nurse practitioners (NPs), those with advanced training who specialize in psychiatric disorders, may be licensed to prescribe anti-depressants and other medications.
PSYCHIATRIC NURSES	A nurse who specializes in psychiatry, in helping those who have mental health problems, may be part of your team on an inpatient unit and in some outpatient centers.

- *Psychiatrists* are medical doctors (MDs or DOs) who are specialty trained, licensed, and board certified to treat mental illnesses such as major depression, bipolar disorder, anxiety, and other conditions. They are the mental health providers who evaluate your family member and prescribe medications such as antidepressants.
- *Clinical psychologists* are master's degree or PhD specialists trained and licensed (PhD) in evaluating and treating mental illnesses using various kinds of talk therapy, or *psychotherapy*. Psychologists are sometimes referred to as *therapists*. Different types of psychotherapy exist, and each has a different focus and purpose. A psychologist will know which type is suitable for your family member or friend. Talk therapy can help your family member cope with his illness, understand himself better, learn healthy ways to manage stress, make sound life decisions, and adjust to major losses and life transitions. Talk therapy can be done in a one-to-one setting or in small groups of people with similar problems.
- *Licensed clinical social workers* (LICSWs or LCSWs) also provide talk therapy to individuals or in groups. They cannot prescribe medications.
- *Nurse practitioners* (NPs), nurses with advanced training, can specialize in psychiatric disorders and are licensed to prescribe antidepressants and other psychiatric medications.

If your family member does not have a PCP or a family doctor who will refer him to a mental health professional, call the patient referral telephone line in the Department of Psychiatry at the local community or university hospital. They can match him with a mental health clinician suited to his symptoms. There are also community mental health clinics, school-based mental health clinics, or mental health professionals available through employer groups. If your loved one finds that he or she cannot afford treatment, more treatment options are presented in chapter 5.

If your family member is active military or a military veteran, he or she is entitled to receive mental health care services through the Veterans Administration (VA) Mental Health System and the Department of Defense (DoD). Many veterans' mental health clinics are scattered throughout the country; these clinics have incorporated peer support services. The Wounded Warrior Project has been designed to help veterans who have physical or mental health problems (including post-traumatic stress) navigate this complex system and find appropriate care. The reality is that the system is backed up, with long waiting periods for an appointment, although efforts are being made to remedy this.

NAMI, the National Alliance on Mental Illness, has local chapters and a beneficial program for military service members and veterans' families and support persons called Homefront. It's a six-week peer-taught educational program, done in person or online, that has shown improvement in empowerment, coping, psychological distress, family functioning, caregiving, and knowledge of mental illness. I encourage you to try it.

> **Your family member will need to interview several mental health professionals to find one who is a good fit for her.**

Some private sector clinics are designed to help veterans. Home Base Program (homebase.org), founded in 2009 by the Red Sox Foundation and Massachusetts General Hospital, works in collaboration with the VA and the DoD to promote the health and wellness of veterans and their families. It has been leading regional and national efforts with a multidisciplinary team of experts who work together to help service members, veterans, and their families heal from the invisible wounds, traumatic brain injury, post-traumatic stress, and related conditions.

The success of your family member's treatment often depends on building a trusting relationship with a therapist or psychiatrist who is a good fit for him. The clinician should be someone your family member can freely speak and get along with. How does your family member find a good psychiatrist or therapist? Once the decision is made that professional help would be valuable, the best way is usually for him to get the names of several mental health providers and meet with each one in person to see how it feels. Encourage him to ask questions of the clinicians he interviews. Does the provider have time to meet with him on a regular basis? Does he take your family's type of insurance?

> **Make a list of questions in advance of the first mental health appointment.**

Many people who have mood disorders want to know about the provider's training, background, and specific area of interest in psychiatry. Does he or she have experience in diagnosing and treating depression or bipolar disorder? Your family member will want to find out whether the clinician is respectful and responsive. Is the clinician someone he feels comfortable talking to and with whom he can work over time? This may take one or more meetings to figure out. That's okay and is expected. Not everyone will be a good match.

Your family member may want to know whether the provider has flexible office hours and can accommodate his work or school schedule. He may also be interested in the provider's method of payment and whether his health insurance will cover it. He will want to make sure the mental health clinician will coordinate his care with his PCP. To get the most from his treatment, it is usually recommended that your family member follow all treatment recommendations as prescribed, keep scheduled appointments, arrive to the session sober, be open and honest with the provider, pay attention to the conversation, and do the homework assignments.

Team Approach

The treatment approach that has shown the greatest success and level of satisfaction is one where there is a team of outpatient providers caring for your loved one. This includes his primary care physician in addition to mental health specialists (psychiatrist for medication management, clinical psychologist or social worker for talk therapy, perhaps a social worker for psychosocial issues). Other medical specialists contribute as needed (oncologist, cardiologist, etc). Inpatient psychiatric providers are involved if admission is required. It is a collaborative effort where the team members (who do not have to be in the same place—it can be virtual) communicate regularly with each other about the emotional and physical health of your loved one. This ensures that the most effective mental health treatment with minimal physical consequences or side effects is offered to the person. The collaborative team has been referred to as the person's "pit crew" by Dr. Michael Sharpe, President of the Academy of Consultation-Liaison Psychiatry (personal communication, 2019).

If your loved one is in crisis and unable to think clearly, is psychotic (has lost touch with reality), or is suicidal, his mental health care team will decide the course of his initial treatment. This is for his safety. Otherwise, expect that he will be an active participant working with his mental health provider in a collaborative process called *shared decision making*.

Shared Decision Making

Shared decision making—the model of patient-centered care—is a process in which your loved one and the clinician work together to make decisions and to select diagnostic tests, treatments, and care plans based on clinical evidence while balancing the risks and benefits with his individual (and informed) preferences and values. His provider will clearly, understandably, and respectfully explain several reasonable treatment options. Then your family member and the provider will work together to answer his questions and to help him understand his treatment options. Through this process your loved one will create his preferences based on accurate information.

In some situations, your loved one may use decision aids, or decision tools, to gain additional, reliable information and help him to understand his alternatives. The Mayo Clinic Shared Decision Making National Resource Center (https://shareddecisions.mayoclinic.org) has a simple decision aid called Depression Medication Choice. Its purpose is to provide your family member with additional information about medications and is not meant to be a substitute for consultation with his clinician.

> Shared decision making gives your loved one control over what happens to him.

In the process of shared decision making, your loved one will discuss the things that are important to him, such as his preferences, goals, and values. He will be able to ask and answer certain questions, including whether he is okay with taking medications, or would he prefer to try to avoid them if possible? Is he concerned about particular side effects? Is he willing to change his daily routine or lifestyle to a healthier one to manage his depression? What are the benefits of one treatment over another? What really matters to *him*? What are his treatment goals?

Once that is done to your family member's satisfaction and all of his questions have been answered, he will have a chance to think and consider the pros, cons, and outcomes. Then together they decide on the best treatment approach and build an effective treatment plan that suits his needs and preferences. This is shared decision making.

Why would your loved one want to do this? First, most people are not aware of the many different treatment options available, and shared decision making educates and empowers your loved one to make a choice that best suits him. It gives him a sense of control. The more he understands his options, the better the chance he will follow through on the treatment recommendations. The process of shared decision making takes into account your family member's preferences and values. If your loved one is not well informed about the details necessary to make his decision, he will be unable to assess "what is important to me" and to determine his true preferences. Informed decisions are an optimal goal because the decisions made are better understood, his expectations will be more accurate, and they are more consistent with his personal preferences. His voice is heard; he has input and feels respected. It also helps to build a trusting relationship with his provider and improves satisfaction levels. If he encounters a mental health provider who is not willing to share in the decision-making process, he may want to look for another clinician who will participate.

Is shared decision making hard to do? Most people welcome the opportunity to participate in their care, but there are a few challenges to consider in shared decision making. Those who have low health literacy or difficulty assessing numbers and risk might have a harder time since it's not within their comfort zone. However, it's not impossible. Those persons who come from a cultural background that lacks a tradition in which individuals make their own decisions might find it new and awkward at first. With good communication between provider and your family member, this awkwardness can be overcome.

Shared decision making is the model of patient-centered care.

Jack's story illustrates the value and impact on treatment shared decision making on a person's illness. It shows us how respect for and attention to the person's desires and preferences can lead to improved cooperation with the treatment plan and in turn an improved outcome.

Jack is a 21-year-old young man who became bothered by fatigue, with difficulty sleeping and concentrating in college. Back at home for summer vacation, his symptoms became more pronounced. He was tired and irritable, not interested in any friends or activities, and lost about 15 pounds without trying. His family brought him to their family doctor, who did an evaluation, diagnosed depression and prescribed an antidepressant medication, a plan Jack understood and agreed to.

Jack returned to school in September, and soon his symptoms worsened, with extreme fatigue and trouble with focus and concentration on his studies. At Thanksgiving, his parents were concerned about the downward course of his illness but because he was now over 21 they could not force him into treatment or discuss that treatment with his doctors. They encouraged him to see his PCP again, who then arranged for Jack to see a psychiatrist for medication management and a clinical psychologist for talk therapy.

Jack resisted at first. He did not know what to expect and didn't want his friends to find out. But he went to see his providers anyway and asked a lot of questions. He told them he didn't like his first antidepressant medication because it made him feel groggy. He wanted to resume his life and activities with friends, sports, playing the guitar, and continuing his education. He has always been an active, athletic, fairly private guy and was concerned about being forced to talk about his "feelings." Jack was satisfied with their answers to his questions and concerns and their thoughtful approach. He really liked that they spoke with him privately, not just with his parents, and asked about what was important to him. He was impressed that he was asked about his priorities, preferences, goals, and values and that his preferences were respected. Over time, he felt comfortable with and agreed to the proposed treatment plan. Jack has continued in therapy for the past six months, is making good progress, and plans to finish his education next year. He will keep in contact with his outpatient mental health providers with student health services as a backup.

Treatment Contract

While in treatment your loved one may be asked to create a Treatment Contract with his provider, sometimes known as an Action Plan for Relapse Prevention (Noonan 2013). There are several versions of a treatment contract now available. This simple document used by many in psychiatry is an agreement that the person who has depression or bipolar disorder creates with his therapist or psychiatrist. It identifies his or her treatment team, his unique triggers and warning signs for worsening mood disorder, the steps to take that have been helpful in the past, the things he will and will not do in response to worsening symptoms, and descriptions of how others can help. It can be quite useful. A sample blank form is found in table 4.2.

Psychiatric Advance Directive

A Psychiatric Advance Directive (PAD) is a legal document that your loved one creates in which he or she details specific instructions for her mental health care in a future situation when, due to illness, she is not considered competent to make her own health care decisions. It is written at a time when things are stable and well, before the anticipated need. A PAD is an important way for providers and family members to understand what she would like to have happen so that you can best advocate for her. The document is used when the person who created it experiences an acute episode of a psychiatric illness and becomes unable to make or communicate decisions about her treatment. The PAD helps to lessen the tension around an inpatient admission and helps to make it a more positive experience. The provider keeps a copy of the signed form in the person's medical record, and the person keeps a copy where it is easily available, such as taped to the refrigerator.

A PAD is a legal form that needs to be witnessed or signed by a notary as required by state law. It's a document that is recognized by about one-half of the states in the United States. Each PAD is individualized, reflecting the person's preferences and expectations. An example of the things it might include are listed in appendix B at the back of this book.

| TABLE 4.2. **Action Plan for Relapse Prevention** |

When I'm feeling well I . . .
Describe your baseline

To stay well, every day I need to . . .

MY TRIGGERS
Events and situations that can cause an increase in your symptoms

TABLE 4.2. **Action Plan for Relapse Prevention** (*continued*)

MY WARNING SIGNS

A change in thoughts, feelings, behaviors, routine, or self-care noticed by yourself or others that are different from your baseline.

ACTIONS to take in Response to Warning Signs

What can I do when I first notice the signs?

Signature (patient): _____ Date: _____

Signature (provider): _____ Date: _____

TABLE 4.2. **Action Plan for Relapse Prevention** (*continued*)

ACTION PLAN

Plan for when symptoms are worse, when you notice your Warning Signs

Things I will do . . .

☐ Contact my doctor(s) early:

Psychiatrist _____ tel#: _____

Psychologist/therapist _____ tel#: _____

Other _____ tel#: _____

☐ Treat any physical medical problems.

☐ Attend to self-care and routine, even if don't feel like it.

☐ Get enough sleep and balanced meals (nutrition).

☐ Take medications as prescribed. Note any recent medication changes.

☐ NO alcohol or drugs.

☐ Other

Supportive persons I will contact and involve (friends, family) . . .

1. _____ tel#: _____

2. _____ tel#: _____

3. _____ tel#: _____

4. _____ tel#: _____

5. _____ tel#: _____

TABLE 4.2. **Action Plan for Relapse Prevention** (*continued*)

Things I will do (coping strategies) to manage or that provide soothing and distraction . . .

1.

2.

3.

4.

5.

Things I will NOT do . . .

1.

2.

3.

Other people can help me by . . .

1.

2.

3.

Signature (patient): _____ Date: _____

Signature (provider): _____ Date: _____

TYPES OF TREATMENT

When considering professional treatment for any mental health condition, keep in mind that there is no quick fix or magic pill to whisk away your loved one's emotional pain. It most likely took a long time for him to get to this place and will take a while for him to understand and unravel it. Treatment requires a lot of hard work and can feel frustrating at times. Therapy sessions can open painful wounds that can create dread and anxiety and be too raw and difficult sometimes, with discomfort that might last for days or weeks afterward. Medications take weeks before any signs of improvement are obvious, which requires extraordinary patience. Your job is to be as encouraging as possible and to point out moments of progress in your loved one.

> The most effective therapy often involves a combination of medication and talk therapy.

Various types of therapy have proven effective for people who have depression. The most effective kind depends on the person's symptoms, medical history, and, to some extent, the type of therapy (if any) he has had in the past. Sometimes medication alone is sufficient, sometimes talk therapy alone is sufficient, and sometimes a combination is needed. It can be difficult to predict how any one person will respond to treatment. She may have to try several medications or types of treatment before finding the most effective one for her needs. The most effective therapy, in all but the earliest forms of depression, often involves working with both a psychiatrist for medication and a therapist for talk therapy.

Talk Therapy

Talk therapy, or psychotherapy, is a type of guided therapeutic conversation that focuses on a person's psychological and emotional problems, distorted thinking, and troublesome behaviors. It can help her cope with her illness, understand herself better, learn healthy ways to manage stress, make sound life decisions, and adjust to major life losses and transitions. Talk therapy can be done one-to-one or in a group setting.

One common and effective type of talk therapy is called *Cognitive Behavioral Therapy*, or CBT. This method in psychotherapy is based on the connection between our thoughts, feelings, and actions. CBT teaches a person to identify and change thinking patterns that may be distorted, beliefs that are inaccurate, and behaviors that are unhelpful.

Mindfulness–based CBT is a somewhat different approach that is also effective for some people. It has a focus of intentionally being in the moment, not dwelling on past or future events.

Dialectical behavior therapy (DBT), another type of psychotherapy, teaches concrete cognitive behavioral and mindfulness skills in four modules: (1) mindfulness, (2) interpersonal effectiveness, (3) emotional regulation, and (4) distress tolerance. The skills learned in DBT can help a person deal with issues in a more balanced, less disruptive and irritable manner. DBT has been shown to be an effective additional therapy to antidepressant medication, resulting in improvement in depressive symptoms.

Behavioral Activation

Loss of interest in the activities a person once enjoyed, or anhedonia, is common in depression. This leads to him stop doing those things because he or she thinks it's not worth the effort; the depression symptoms worsen and he feels more isolated, detached, withdrawn, and anxious. Since it has been observed that one's behavior affects emotions and mood in both a positive and negative way, it's helpful for your loved one to get involved in activities that have the potential to improve his mood. This is the basis of *behavioral activation*, a CBT approach and coping strategy for depression that can positively affect mood, decrease the risk for depression, and help to treat it.

Behavioral activation is a type of behavior therapy often used along with other therapeutic skills and strategies. The aim of behavioral activation is to help a person re-engage in enjoyable, rewarding activities and develop or enhance his problem-solving skills. That will counteract the isolation, withdrawal and avoidance patterns common to depression and in turn improve mood. In addition, doing things that are a little challenging will provide a sense of accomplishment and mastery that may also boost his mood.

Behavioral activation is done with a therapist who helps the person identify goals (pleasurable activities), schedule positive experiences, address the obstacles to achieving them, and improve problem-solving skills. The goals need to be

specific
measurable
attainable
realistic, and
trackable

The person should pursue only those activities that have importance and meaning to him (not something of importance to others or things that he *should* do); go slow and start with the easiest ones first, and then enlist the support of others. Behavioral activation can be difficult to do when a person has low motivation or increased anxiety. This is where the strategy *action precedes motivation* helps.

How does this work for your loved one? Perhaps he is depressed and wants to stay in bed all day, no longer out exercising, something he had enjoyed doing in the past and scolds himself for not doing now. He's full of guilt and excuses at the moment—it's cold, he's tired, he's not interested. The therapist would help him identify one or two types of exercise as a goal for him to participate in, something he likes or used to like doing, that he's skilled at, and is realistic for him to engage in: jogging, swimming, biking, yoga, basketball, whatever. The clinician then helps him identify the obstacles to achieving that goal. Maybe he has fatigue so it's choosing the optimal time of day when he has the most energy, starting slow. Maybe he has trouble with motivation so it's having an exercise partner to whom he'll be accountable for showing up, and who will make it more enjoyable and sociable.

Then they will break the activity down to realistic but not overwhelming small steps at first. He might begin with doing a series of small skills drills or doing the activity two to three times a week for 15 minutes at a time, increasing in time and intensity. Once obstacles have been identified and addressed and the initial steps identified, then together they will identify ways to monitor and track his activity—either with a journal, a log, or an electronic device—so that he can appreciate his participation and progress, track improvement in mood, and make modifications to more challenging activities as required. The therapist will be there to review his experience and help him make adaptive changes as needed.

Virtual Visits

For people who live in rural areas, access to mental health professionals is often a problem. Few mental health providers may be available, and they are often a great distance away. Sometimes their schedules are overbooked because of the need to cover large geographic areas.

One recent option is a *virtual visit*—or an online appointment similar to Skype or FaceTime—called telemedicine. This term is often confused with telehealth, which is a general term for a broad array of technologies and tactics that deliver virtual medical visits as well as other health services and health education. While Medicare has authorized telehealth for certain medical visits, a virtual visit for mental health may or may not be the best option for your loved one. A virtual visit can be a good and effective experience for patient and provider. However, it may not lend itself optimally to the care of someone who has a mood disorder or other psychiatric illness; it may miss a thorough observation of the person and whether he has impaired gait or unsteadiness, signs of alcoholic breath and certain diagnostic body odors. Reimbursement for telemedicine and telehealth varies, but it may be covered by health insurance. There are licensure issues when care is provided across states. And there are significant privacy concerns. Another issue is that virtual visits do not allow for the patient-therapist relationship to truly develop. That bond is the key to successful therapeutic treatment, and without a private, safe place in which to communicate openly, therapy is jeopardized. Virtual visits may be useful as a tool to use in-between face-to-face appointments with an established mental health provider who already knows your loved one or if he lives in a remote geographic area; research on this is ongoing.

Medications

Many different types of medications can be used to treat depression (see appendix A). The choice of medication is based on your loved one's particular combination of depression symptoms. It may take several weeks, or months, to see the effects. That can be frustrating and requires realistic expectations and a lot of patience on everybody's part. The greatest challenge for your loved one is the ability to tolerate the unbearable symptoms of depression while waiting for the treatment or medications to work.

At times, more than one antidepressant is required, or a switch to another category of antidepressant is indicated based on the person's response and set of symptoms. Often another medication (which is not an antidepressant) is added to assist the initial antidepressant in working more effectively; this is called *augmentation*. For example, thyroid medication, atypical antipsychotics, and some herbal supplements may be used for this purpose.

Recently, there have been trials using ketamine for depression in special circumstances. Ketamine is a medication sometimes used for anesthesia that also has been misused as a street drug of abuse (Special-K). However, in small doses, it can be helpful for depression in *some* people. In March 2019, the Food and Drug Administration approved a special form of ketamine for use in depression, a nasal spray called *Esketamine*, used two to three times per week. It is administered under a clinician's direct observation because confusion may occur in the first two hours after taking it; the confusion clears rapidly, and then your loved one goes home. For all medications, each person has a different experience.

Treatment for bipolar disorder is different. Antidepressant medications should not be used for bipolar depression, as they make the condition worse. Recommended treatment for bipolar disorder (those diagnosed over time with both mania and depression) includes a mood stabilizer alone or combined with an atypical antipsychotic drug, along with psychotherapy. Commonly used mood stabilizers are lithium (Escalate or Lithobid), valproic acid (Depakote or Depakene), carbamazapene (Tegretol), and lamotrigine (Lamictal). Antipsychotics include olanzapine (Zyprexa), risperidone (Risperdal), quetiapine (Seroquel), aripiprazole (Abilify), brexpiprazole (Rexulti), and lurasidone (Latuda). Food and Drug Administration–approved treatments for bipolar depression are a Zyprexa-Prozac combination, Seroquel, Latuda, Lamictal, and electroconvulsive therapy (ECT). Know that the Zyprexa/Prozac combination and Seroquel can cause metabolic syndrome (see chapter 1), a physiologic problem of central weight gain and obesity, increased lipids, high blood pressure, and increased risk of diabetes. A preferred starting combination for bipolar depression has been found to be lithium and Lamictal (Nierenberg 2018).

> Medications and psychotherapy (talk therapy) complement each other.

Medication therapy and psychotherapy alone are each effective in treating depression and reducing the risk of relapse and recurrence. In combination, they offer an even greater benefit against relapse, or a return of symptoms. Psychotherapy offers a broader range of benefits than antidepressants do, such as improving your loved one's level of functioning, diminishing residual symptoms, targeting specific symptoms (such as guilt, hopelessness, and pessimism), teaching coping skills and improving interpersonal relationships. The effects of psychotherapy are longer lasting and sustained beyond the end of treatment.

Somatic Treatments

Somatic treatments are physically applied to the body and have an effect on the brain; several are described here. One treatment option sometimes offered when medications do not work well or cannot be used for medical reasons is *electroconvulsive therapy*, or ECT (also called *shock therapy*). This treatment is given in the hospital, either as an inpatient or outpatient procedure. Your family member may go home after a few hours. First, your family member or friend receives a short-acting anesthesia medication to put him to sleep for a few minutes. A very brief, very low electric current is sent to the brain through *electrodes*, small sticky pads, which are placed on his scalp. Electrodes transmit the current to the mood center of his brain.

It may sound scary, but ECT does not hurt, and your family member is unaware of the process. Some people may have a mild headache for a few hours afterward. Others may lose a portion of their memory for around the time of the treatment; for example, they can't remember whether they brushed their teeth that morning! ECT is usually given three times a week for several weeks. Most people find their depression symptoms improve noticeably after the first few treatments.

Another proven effective treatment in some people who have depression is *repetitive transcranial magnetic stimulation* (rTMS). This procedure uses a magnetic field to stimulate nerve cells in certain areas of the brain. rTMS involves placing a special wand, or magnetic coil, on a precise spot on the scalp. The coil directs magnetic pulses to a portion of the brain involved in mood regulation. Each treatment typically lasts for 40 minutes, five times a week for four to six weeks and then is tapered to twice a week for three weeks.

The dose and position on the scalp are individualized for each person. (The dose is determined by the strength, pattern, and duration of the magnetic pulse.) Several different types of coils are designed to deliver a localized magnetic field in a specific pattern and frequency (in continuous or burst patterns): the timing and length of treatment is slightly different for each of these. rTMS does not require anesthesia, and there is no confusion or memory loss afterward. There may be a mild headache and scalp tingling. Many who have used this treatment have found improvement in their depression symptoms. Various other treatments are currently being studied for their effectiveness.

Support Groups

Often, individuals who receive treatment for depression find it helpful to speak with others experiencing the same symptoms. Support groups around the country exist just for this purpose. The outpatient psychiatry department at a hospital or patient (consumer) organizations such as the Depression and Bipolar Support Alliance (DBSA) or NAMI usually sponsor them. The national organizations have local chapters and are open to everyone. These organizations also have sections for friends and family members seeking support. NAMI conducts a training program for families. Family to Family is a 12-week course on accepting and supporting those with mental illness. Approximately 300,000 people have taken it so far and have given excellent feedback.

Inpatient Care

Occasionally, someone who has depression or bipolar disorder is too ill to manage at home or go to outpatient therapy appointments. She may also feel unsafe or suicidal. This situation can overwhelm you as a caretaker. Most people in your position cannot manage this alone.

In this case, your family member needs treatment in the inpatient psychiatry unit of a hospital. Inpatient care is a more intense form of treatment, where she receives daily individual and group therapy as well as medication management. An inpatient unit provides a safe environment during a rough time. This is especially important for those who have disorganized or suicidal thoughts.

If you believe that your loved one is too ill to manage at home, your first response is to call or encourage her to call her psychiatrist or psychologist, who will arrange for evaluation and a hospital admission. If she has not yet established a mental health provider, your best options are to contact her PCP or take her to your local Emergency Department, where they will evaluate her and make the necessary arrangements.

> Inpatient care
> can be lifesaving.

Being in the hospital can frighten some people at first, especially when the person does not feel well and does not know what to expect, but most leave the hospital feeling better. Most people treated in a hospital find it to be extremely helpful and even lifesaving.

Once in the hospital, she will be cared for by a treatment team that usually consists of a senior (attending) psychiatrist, nurse, and social worker. If she is in a teaching hospital of a university medical center, she will usually have a psychiatry resident and perhaps a medical student attending to her. She may also see a clinical psychologist. The inpatient unit will focus on her safety and provide for her daily needs. The treatment team's role is to see her each day, to review her current treatment plan and suggest modifications as required, and to encourage her to attend group therapy sessions with other inpatients. The inpatient treatment plan is a collaborative plan between your loved one and the team. She has the right to decide what feels appropriate and helpful for her and to accept or reject their assessment and recommendations, as long as her decisions are safe.

Admission to an inpatient psychiatry unit can last 7 to 10 days or longer, depending on the needs of your family member and her response to initial treatment. The team will be in contact with her outpatient providers, if she has already established them. If she has not, the inpatient team will recommend and arrange for a mental health professional, someone who is covered by her insurance plan and located in her area, for her to see following discharge from the hospital. Discharge plans are very specific, detailing any changes in her medications and treatment plan that your family member agrees to. She will leave the hospital with written instructions and specific appointments already lined up, including what to do if problems arise.

WHEN SOMEONE REFUSES TREATMENT

Some people have a hard time accepting treatment for depression. Your family member or friend may not believe that treatment will help him, may not recognize the need for treatment, or may just plain refuse to go. If you talk him into going, he may go—but unwillingly.

He might also reject offers of help from anyone. Here are some phrases you may be familiar with: "Get off my back." "Nothing anyone can do will help." "Nobody understands." Knowing that someone needs treatment but encountering their strong resistance to it can put you in a difficult position.

Unfortunately, you'll find no easy answers or concrete solutions for this one—no magic solutions, clinical trials, or official guidelines from academic societies (except in cases of crisis). There are only suggestions based on families' experiences. Families struggle tremendously to convince their loved ones to seek treatment. It is one of the most difficult things people face. Adults have a right to decide for themselves what treatment they receive and what happens to them and have the right to refuse treatment. If your family member does not perceive the need for treatment, the conversation becomes one sided.

Reasons for Refusing Treatment

Why would someone who desperately needs treatment refuse it? There are several reasons. Your family member or friend may believe that seeking help from a mental health professional means he's a failure. It's hard for someone who has always been able to deal with his own problems to accept help. It may make him feel vulnerable and inadequate. And because of the distorted, negative thinking common in depression, he may perceive any efforts to help as intrusive.

Your family member or friend who has depression may be concerned about the financial burden of receiving treatment. Or his main concern may be privacy issues: he could be afraid that if his friends, coworkers, or employer find out, he'll lose his job, his reputation, or those close to him. He might fear being judged unfairly, criticized, or negatively labeled because of his illness and cut off socially. This is known as the *stigma* of mental illness.

Your family member may also believe that treatment is not effective—at least for him. He may fear becoming dependent on or addicted to medications, dread the side effects they can create, or believe that psychiatric drugs will change who he is. He might also believe the rumors that he will feel like a "zombie" or lose his creativity on medications. Media reports about the adverse effects of medications and negative television advertisements can also contribute to fears about treatment.

> Help your loved one understand the reasons he might be refusing treatment.

Perhaps your loved one is afraid of the strong emotions that treatment may bring up. This is a common fear in people with mood disorders. Maybe his concerns are based on mistaken beliefs about depression and its treatment.

What Can You Do?

What can you do when your family member or friend rejects your help or refuses to go for treatment? Begin by emphasizing that you love him and are concerned about him. Try to calmly explain exactly what you see in him that is different from his usual self and provide specific examples. Approach the topic by saying, "You seem to be more down than usual in the past few weeks, and I notice you're not sleeping well. I'm concerned about you. I think this may be a good time for you to speak with Dr. Jones. He can help."

Tell him why you think it's important that he seek help. Mention symptoms of depression or bipolar disorder that he has, that they are symptoms of an illness and point out that treatment may help relieve them. Make him aware that these symptoms and his problems will not improve on their own and that some savvy help may be necessary for him to feel better. Emphasize that you're recommending he get treatment for his own health and well-being. It may be the only way he can realize his dreams of finishing school, getting back to work, enjoying himself with friends—whatever parts of life he's missing out on. You might mention that having an evaluation doesn't mean he has to decide on or agree to treatment; seeing treatment as an option rather than a foregone conclusion may make him feel more inclined to go. Try to be firm, steady, and persistent.

If misinformation about mood disorders and treatment is behind his reluctance to see a mental health professional, provide him with accurate information about his illness. Once you know his concerns, you or his PCP can address those worries with facts. Gaining information is a powerful tool to counteract resistance. Having knowledge about his illness makes things less scary and may help reverse your family member's resistance to treatment.

He might just feel fatigued and overwhelmed by the idea of seeing a mental health professional. This is where you can help by calling to schedule appointments and arrange health insurance coverage, if required. Search out the names of a few mental health providers in your area and let him decide which ones he will interview. If he's anxious about going the first few times, offer to go along and sit in the waiting room. You might suggest that he prepare for the appointment by organizing his questions and issues on paper or on a smartphone ahead of time. Do whatever you can to discourage his excuses, remove any obstacles, and make it easier for him to go.

> **Point out what is different today from her usual baseline self.**

You cannot force an adult into treatment unless he is in crisis or, in the rare case, you need to take legal steps to ensure his safety. For example, in the extremely ill, this might mean getting a court order to ensure he takes his medications. While it's difficult to do, respect his right to refuse your help or treatment *unless* you believe he could harm himself or others. Then you must call for professional help or dial 9-1-1 immediately, regardless of his preferences.

For adolescents. Parents or guardians can try to use their influence to get an adolescent into treatment. This may be easier said than done. He or she can give you a really hard time about not wanting to go. This issue is the cause of many family disruptions. You may have to adopt a *tough love* approach. Highlight that you're motivated by your love and concern for him. Getting him to stay in therapy may be quite another challenge, influenced in part by his relationship with the therapist and the traits of his age group. Try to give your adolescent a sense of personal control by allowing him to make some of the (minor) decisions about his treatment. This has been an effective strategy in many families. In addition, emphasize that treatment may help him reach some of the goals he's been talking about.

If the person who has depression is a young adult, a spouse, a sibling, or a parent, your options are more limited. You cannot force a child over age 18 or other family members to seek treatment. His medical encounters are private, and you have limited access to speak with his health care providers. This is to respect his privacy. Use the strength of your personal connection with him and gentle pressure from other family members to persuade him to seek treatment. A family meeting with his health care provider may finally convince him.

There is one thing you can try if he has previously been in treatment and is now experiencing a relapse or recurrence. Encourage him to adopt the terms of a Treatment Contract, or Action Plan for Relapse Prevention, with his mental health provider. This is *his* plan, described earlier in this chapter that outlines what to do when the warning signs of worsening mood symptoms occur. You may have some success in getting your family member to abide by his own words in this document and in this way return to treatment.

> Focus your comments on your family member's strengths and positive qualities.

For seniors. If your family member who has depression is elderly, you may need to focus on his safety. This is particularly true if he lives alone or with an elderly spouse or seems confused. In some cases, he may not remember to take medications as prescribed or may not care. He may not be steady enough to care for himself. The loneliness and chronic medical problems of people in this age group put them at high risk for suicide. When you are not available, another family member or an outside "sitter" may need to be present at all times until the situation improves. (A sitter is someone who you hire to be present 24/7, in shifts, to observe, assist and keep your loved one safe.)

Try not to take your loved one's resistance to therapy—and to your own efforts to help him—personally. You may feel resentful, angry, or frustrated, as these are natural responses to the situation. Use some of the coping strategies outlined in chapter 9 to ease these moments. Take a deep breath, go for a walk, talk to a friend, or get professional help yourself. This can be in individual therapy or by going to a support group for family members. Coping in this situation means paying attention to your feelings, managing your stress, and getting the help *you* need, too.

Paying for Mental Health Treatment

HEALTH INSURANCE BASICS

One question that often haunts those who have a family member with a mood disorder is, "How is my loved one going to pay for all of these specialized mental health care services?" There's a lot involved, beginning with an initial psychiatric evaluation, psychologic testing as indicated, regular follow-up appointments with a psychiatrist for medication management, and frequent appointments with a clinical psychologist, licensed clinical social worker, or mental health counselor for psychotherapy (talk therapy). Perhaps he or she will see a psychiatric nurse practitioner at some point or join a support or psychoeducational group. Occasionally, she might see others in consultation or for specific neuropsychiatric testing.

If she lives outside of the United States, she may likely reside in a country that has universal health care coverage and be eligible for that. Some nations are more comprehensive than others in what they offer; there is a range of different services. The federal government of Canada funds universal health care coverage for its citizens. The provinces and territories are then mandated to provide coverage for those health care services deemed to be "medically necessary." In some situations, the definition of medical necessity is disputed. The Canadian government pays all mental health–related inpatient and psychiatrist's care, while the majority of mental health outpatient and psychologists visits are either out-of-pocket or paid by third-party insurance. The result is unfortunately long waiting times for a psychotherapy appointment.

Many European nations also have versions of universal health care, with gaps in services in some places, such as for mental and behavioral health and substance use disorder services. The United Kingdom has a universal state-funded health care system, with private health care in a small niche market. From my comparative research, Switzerland appears to have superb coverage, as does France, Norway, Luxembourg, and several others. Germany has a social health insurance system with community-based mental health centers. The government in China covers services they deem necessary, while India has a private health care system with the government covering those below the poverty level. However, having health care coverage does not always translate into having mental health care coverage.

> There is a wide range in the definition of "medical necessity."

Australia has a system where the roles and responsibilities for mental health services are divided and funded among the Australian government, state and territory, and private or non-government sector. With the Australian Institute of Health and Welfare (https://www.aihw.gov.au/reports/mental-health-services/mental-health-services-in-australia/report-contents/summary), the state and territory governments fund and deliver public sector mental health services using specialists in the public acute and psychiatric hospitals and outpatient setting, community mental health care services, and state and territory residential facilities. The government funds services through a Medicare Benefits Schedule and Pharmaceutical Benefits Scheme and supports programs and services (income support, social and community support, disability, workforce participation, housing assistance). The private sector administers mental health services in private psychiatric hospitals and outpatient settings using private health insurance funds.

Health insurance coverage in the United States is complex. Several types of insurance are available to individuals and families:

- Private insurance: purchased individually or through an employer
- Medicaid (government plan for low-income persons and some nursing home care, administered separately by each state)
- Medicare (federal government plan for seniors with limited nursing home care and certain diagnoses like end-stage renal disease (kidney failure) and kidney dialysis
- Medicare Part A: hospital/facility insurance (inpatient)
- Medicare Part B: medical insurance (outpatient, labs)
- Medicare Part D: drugs, prescription medications
- Supplemental Medicare Plan: a plan one purchases separately to fill in the gaps of what is not covered by Part B
- Medicare Advantage: a plan one purchases that combines coverage of the gaps in Parts B and D (a type of supplemental plan)
- CHIP (Children's Health Insurance Plan): government plan for children for those in the low-income group who earn too much to be eligible for Medicaid; administered by the states
- TRICARE and VA Health Care: for active service members, their families, and veterans

Private insurance in the United States can be purchased individually or through an employer group. There are certain rules that apply to employer-based health care plans, depending on their size. What the plans will cover varies based on how the employer group negotiates with the health insurance company. For example, each insurance company (such as Blue Cross, Kaiser, or Cigna) will differ in the kinds of plans they offer, and within those insurance companies, each plan also varies, depending on how well the specific employer group negotiated with them. Each insurance company or employer-based plan within an insurance company does not cover the same services, list of providers, or medications.

Private health insurance in the United States typically involves some kind of cost-sharing between the subscriber (your loved one) and the health insurance company, also known as out-of-pocket spending, which is in addition to paying the health insurance premium. The fees for private health insurance differ under each plan and can add up quickly. Your loved one may face paying the following health costs:

- *Deductible*: the amount a person must pay each year before the insurance plan begins to cover most services (for example, he may pay $1,000 per year before his services are then covered)
- *Co-pay*: a fixed-dollar amount paid per visit, admission, or prescription medication (for example, your loved one would pay $20 per visit each time)
- *Coinsurance*: a percentage of the allowed charge paid for a visit, admission, or prescription medication (for example, he would pay 20% of an allowed prescription drug cost each time)

If your loved one has employer-based private health insurance or is self-employed, these fees are set by the terms of the employer's contract with the health insurance company. Typically, the subscriber (your loved one) pays all three fees; the exact amount will vary based on the contract. If she has employer-based private health insurance and loses her job (is laid off or fired), she has the option of extending her current health plan for up to 18 months under COBRA (Consolidated Omnibus Budget Reconciliation Act), a federal law passed in 1985 that provides for continuing group health insurance coverage for some employees and their families after a job loss or other qualifying event. She must apply for this right away. COBRA may not apply if her employer has fewer than 20 employees. Under COBRA, she will have to pay 100 percent of the insurance premium, but that is less expensive than if she were to go out and buy a new plan on her own. Keep in mind that she has 60 days to enroll in a new plan. If she delays longer than 62 days, she will be subject to an exclusion of preexisting conditions, and her mental illness diagnosis may very likely not be covered by the new plan.

If your loved one is unemployed, he may be able to get an affordable health insurance plan through the Marketplace (see Affordable Care Act), with savings based on his income and household size. He may also qualify for free or low-cost coverage through Medicaid or the Children's Health Insurance Program (CHIP).

Medicare and Medicaid are federal US programs created in 1965 as an amendment to the Social Security Act. They were designed to offer health insurance protection to the elderly, the poor, and people who have disabilities. Medicare, the program for the elderly and people who have disabilities, consists of facility-based care (Part A), physician and provider services (Part B), and prescription drugs (Part D). Medicaid is a joint federal and state program that pays for acute care for the poor as well as long-term care in nursing homes. Relevant to the delivery of mental health care, it includes nonphysician services, services in freestanding outpatient clinics, case management, rehabilitation, and home health care.

The following is important for you to know in general and to help you understand your family member's coverage rights. It applies in *most* cases.

Historically, insurance companies were allowed to offer different types of coverage for mental health and behavioral health as compared with physical health (medical and surgical needs) within the same plan. Then, in 2008, a federal mental health "parity law" was passed in the United States that required, *in most cases*, that mental health and substance use disorders services coverage *must be comparable* to medical/surgical coverage. This is the Paul Wellstone and Pete Domenici Mental Health Parity and Addiction Equity Act and is meant to protect those who have a mental illness, including addictions.

The parity law requires insurance companies to treat mental health, behavioral health, and substance use disorders with coverage equal to (or better than) physical medical coverage (medical and surgical coverage). This means, for example, that the co-pays will be the same for a primary care physician and a psychiatrist's visit (financial equity) and that nonfinancial treatment limits (limits placed on the number of psychiatric visits allowed per year) are eliminated. However, insurance companies can still put treatment limits in place if they are related to "medical necessity" for either psychiatry or medical/surgical visits *as they define it.*

And even though the federal parity law applies to all diagnoses, *insurance plans can still exclude certain mental health diagnoses or medical/surgical diagnoses as they choose.* It all depends on how they define *something.* This can present a major problem if an insurance company defines medical necessity in a nonstandard way or decides to exclude a diagnostic category, and your family member finds himself suddenly not covered for his illness. It's apparently within the law. (Since 2006, Massachusetts is the only state that has universal health insurance coverage.)

> Despite the parity law, insurance plans can still impose treatment limits or exclude certain diagnoses.

The parity law applies to the following conditions:

1. Employer-sponsored plans for companies with more than 51 employees
2. Most group health plans with 50 or fewer employees unless "grandfathered" in
3. Coverage purchased through health exchanges (the Marketplace) created under the Affordable Care Act of 2010
4. Children covered through CHIP who receive an array of full mental and behavioral health services
5. Most Medicaid programs (requirements vary with the program. States determine which services to cover for adults.)

Some government plans and programs are *exempt* from the parity law; the mental health services they cover varies.

1. Medicare
   a. Part A: covers some inpatient mental health services
   b. Part B: covers some outpatient services
   c. Part D: covers some medications—the drug formulary varies.
      Advantage Plan: need to check membership materials for coverage
2. Some state government employer plans (for example, teachers, state university employees; also individual states may opt out)

The parity law *does not require* insurers to provide mental health benefits. It does state that, if mental health benefits are offered, they cannot have more restrictive requirements than the medical/surgical benefits offered by the same plan. Most large group plans already offered mental health benefits before the parity law took effect in 2008.

Affordable Care Act

In 2010, the Patient Protection and Affordable Care Act of 2010 (ACA), commonly known as Obamacare, was passed. It was designed to make health insurance available to more people. The ACA mainly benefits individuals and small groups who pay their own insurance, including those who are uninsured or are low income. The effect of the ACA at 10 years has been to reduce the number of uninsured persons in the United States and to improve access to health care services, especially among low-income persons and those of color. This has translated to improved health status in Americans. Some people have a bad impression of this regulation, mostly because they don't understand it, but I urge you to be open-minded and read on to learn more about it.

The ACA is founded on three principles. First is expansion of Medicaid coverage in low-income persons, making eligibility based on income rather than on individual personal factors like pregnancy, age or disability. Second are subsidies for the purchase of private health insurance for low-income persons who are without access to employer-based programs or other public programs. The person's insurance purchase is done through newly created private individual insurance "marketplaces" or exchanges. Third, the ACA also created some health insurance reform measures, such as eliminating discrimination in persons with preexisting health conditions, requiring all private insurers offer coverage to young adults up to age 26 under their parents plan, and requiring the plans include ten categories of essential and preventive health benefits. It all sounds good, but partisan conflict in Congress has since modified the terms of the original law.

When the ACA began, every person was required to have documented health insurance for 9 out of 12 months of the year or pay a fine or penalty (as an incentive to enroll). In 2019 a new law (Tax Cuts and Jobs Act 2018) was passed so that people no longer have to pay the *federal* penalty if they do not have health insurance. Yet some states still require a person to pay a *state* penalty if they do not have insurance: these include New Jersey, District of Columbia, Massachusetts, Vermont and Rhode Island.

This new (2019) law removed the incentive to enroll and many young, healthy people have chosen to not purchase health insurance, disproportionately leaving the insurance companies with those who have more medical problems. This places a financial burden on the whole system and raises costs.

Here's how the ACA now works. Individuals are obligated to carry health insurance, either through their employers, the ACA Marketplace (Exchange), or individually. The ACA offers premium subsidies (tax credits) for low- and moderate-income persons (those with incomes between 100 and 400 percent of the federal poverty level) to lower the cost and help them buy coverage. Tax credits are not available to those who qualify for Medicaid or CHIP, those covered by Medicare Part A, or those who have employer-sponsored coverage. Under the ACA, health insurance premiums are based on income and location.

The ACA also expands Medicaid eligibility to include those earning up to 138 percent of the federal poverty level and creates a small business insurance Marketplace to help firms with 50 or fewer workers cover their workers. Unfortunately, not all states have chosen to expand Medicaid eligibility; these 14 states are mainly in the southern United States.

ACA requires insurance companies to cover ten (10) essential health benefits that includes mental health, addiction and many preventive services. However, if your plan began before March 2010, it can be "grandfathered" in and will not have to provide these benefits.

The ACA states that health insurance companies cannot exclude those who have preexisting medical conditions (including mental health) or drop those who become sick. A preexisting medical condition is a medical or psychological problem you had before you signed up for that particular insurance plan. The ACA also allows families to include children up to age 26 under a parent's plan.

> The ACA covers those who have preexisting medical conditions.

Under the ACA individuals may purchase health insurance coverage through a state or a federally sponsored health insurance exchange, or the Marketplace, which makes buying easier and more affordable. The exchanges allow people to compare health plans, answer questions, get reduced costs, and enroll in a plan of their choice. You can learn more at HealthCare.gov.

Despite its goal of universal health coverage, the ACA leaves a large number of Americans without access to insurance. Since the ACA went into effect in 2014, those who had no health insurance dropped from 15 percent to 9 percent for all individuals ages 12 and older. The percentage of persons who have a mental disorder and no health insurance fell from 21 percent in 2013 to 12 percent in 2016. Why aren't these number better? The uninsured here represent those with incomes just above 400 percent of the federal poverty level who are not eligible for Medicaid or tax credits, undocumented immigrants, low-income individuals living in states that do not expand Medicaid coverage, and others. Even so, early results suggest that the ACA has improved access to mental health services and has had a modest effect on substance use treatment so far. Having health insurance results in less out-of-pocket spending, increased access to services, and better health outcomes.

The system is not perfect and still has many cracks in it. In some instances, the deductibles and co-payments are high and unaffordable, and your family member may need to register an appeal to the health insurance company. Also, some mental health professionals are not all on the health insurer's "network" (the insurer's list of included providers) and those clinicians who remain may have a schedule that's full to capacity, so they're not taking on new patients. It may take many phone calls or being put on a wait list to get a provider that your family member feels comfortable with. These are all real problems where you can be of help in advocating, making phone calls, and filing complaints and appeals.

If your loved one's mental health care services have been denied by an insurance company, do not just sit back and accept it. Make inquiries and have him or her file an appeal. An appeal is a formal complaint you make to the insurance company about something you believe is not right or appropriate about the insurance coverage or a denial of care. Know that the appeal process is not easy. It is designed to make the person and his doctor jump through hoops or do things required by the insurance company, based on their internal guidelines, that may not be necessarily indicated for all persons clinically. For example, if the provider prescribes a new medication—let's call it medication B—the insurer might require your loved one to try a course of medication A before they authorize his use of medication B even though the doctor might disagree with that decision and sees no clinical reason for doing it. Then your loved one has to file an appeal. Appeals are meant to be difficult, to make your family member and his provider stop trying and give up the fight. I strongly urge you to not give up!

Finding affordable mental health treatment can be challenging for those whose lives are in transition or who have limited health care resources. In the following story about James, we can see several different options for treatment providers in the community that he came to use. While a person who has depression may feel too fatigued and disorganized to seek these out, it's important for you the family members to understand what choices are out there and available to someone who is struggling. Your role may be to help identify these options and let your loved one then decide which course to take.

James is a 24-year-old man who started having symptoms of bipolar disorder in graduate school, when he was diagnosed with an episode of bipolar hypomania. Because of his illness, he has been unable to finish his last two semesters. James first approached his university's health center, which referred him to a psychiatrist for medication treatment and to one of their mental health counselors, a licensed clinical social worker. James seemed to connect fairly well with her, seeing her for a few sessions during his third year. On a visit back home with his parents, his bipolar depression symptoms became more pronounced. He was tearful, fatigued, not interested in any friends or activities, and gained about 12 pounds without trying. James's family brought him to their family doctor, who did

*an evaluation and prescribed an antidepressant medication, which was
not the best choice for someone who has bipolar disorder. .*

*He went back to school the next semester and soon found his depres-
sion symptoms worsening. Eventually, James took a leave of absence from
school, without telling his parents, living in an apartment with his old
roommates. Now out of school and without access to the student health
services, James had no money for treatment. His best friend found him a
community mental health center nearby, and he spoke with a counselor
there over several months. During his next visit with his parents, they
were concerned about James's worsening depression but were aware that
since he was over 21 they could not force him into treatment or discuss
that treatment with his doctors. They encouraged James to return to his
primary care physician again, who then arranged for him to see another
psychiatrist for medication management and a clinical psychologist for
talk therapy.*

*James and his parents were also relieved to find that his mental health
treatment was still covered under their health insurance policy until
age 26 under the ACA (this is specific to the United States and is not an
issue in other countries). He has continued with this treatment plan for
the past six months, is making good progress, and will return to school
next semester. James will continue treatment with his outpatient mental
health providers and is reassured to have the referral from student health
services as needed.*

WHAT TO DO WHEN YOUR FAMILY MEMBER CAN'T AFFORD TREATMENT

Health care is expensive. If you live in a country that offers wide-ranging
health care coverage, including mental health services, you are fortunate.
Despite the foundations of the ACA, more and more people in the United
States find they are unable to afford professional mental health services.
Some become unemployed due to their illness and then lose their more
comprehensive health care benefits; many others work part time in a job
that just does not offer any health care coverage at all. Or there may be insurance limits placed on the number of services a person can receive, thus
raising his out-of-pocket expenses. Savings, which are sometimes meager,
dwindle. If any of this is true for your family member or friend, what are his
options? Here are a few ideas:

- *In-training programs* at university teaching hospitals, where clinical care is provided by residents-in-training who are supervised by senior psychiatry staff members.
- *Sliding scale clinics* where the fee for mental health services is adjusted on a sliding scale for those who have documented financial need.
- *Pro bono (free)* care offered by some mental health professionals—this care depends on the individual provider, and eligibility varies.
- *School clinics*, where mental health care, usually short term, is provided by counselors in high schools and colleges, often for free or at a reduced rate.
- *Community services*, such as mental health clinics offered by state, federal, and local health departments for those in financial need (see a list of these at Centers for Disease Control and Prevention website, CDC.gov).
- *Referral to low-cost services* through NAMI (National Alliance on Mental Illness) website (www.NAMI.org) or by calling 800-950-6264.
- *Listing of free mental health clinics* provided by SAMHSA (Substance Abuse and Mental Health Services Administration) at SAMHSA.gov.
- *Employment-based Employee Assistance Programs* (EAPs) provide mental health services to employees for free (for several sessions) or at a reduced rate—check with your employer.
- The *National Suicide Prevention Lifeline* at 800-273-8255 offers emergency assessment.

Medications can be very expensive, and not all are covered, especially if you have a marginal health insurance plan. There are some ways to get a financial exemption from the pharmaceutical companies (drug manufacturers) for low-cost or free medications for those who meet certain income requirements. You will have to contact each company and apply to them directly if your loved one meets their criteria.

6

Challenges in Caring for Someone Who Has a Mood Disorder

Most people who have depression don't experience this illness alone. They have family members and close friends, like you, who care and want to know what they can do to help. Depression and bipolar disorder are considered family illnesses for two main reasons. First, mood disorders can be genetic, or run in families. Second, it usually affects a person's friends or family in some negative way. You and other family members may feel emotionally down, put off, shut out, worn out, or guilty from dealing with a mood disorder in your loved one 24 hours a day. You may feel you've done something to cause her unhappiness, isolation, or irritability.

You may find that your family plans are frequently interrupted, personal finances are affected, and more of your energy goes toward dealing with your loved one's life issues. It can be exhausting. There may be more stress in the family in having to cope with a member who is ill. The family may experience added burdens as health insurers and HMOs fail to fully understand the person's medical needs and the level of required care. The financial strain of paying for mental health services is significant.

> Depression and bipolar disorder affect the whole family.

It is not easy to help someone with any medical problem, including a mental health disorder like depression and bipolar disorder. It's difficult for caregivers in your position to find the balance between providing much-needed help to a family member and supporting her sense of independence. While you want to help, at the same time, you don't want to incapacitate her by taking over her activities of daily living (laundry, phone calls, meals, other responsibilities). You may feel burned out from the work and effort if the illness lasts a long time. Most important, helping someone who has a mood disorder is and feels different from caring for a person who has other medical problems. It carries with it special challenges.

Lack of insight. Very often the person who has a mood disorder is unaware that what he is experiencing is actually a set of symptoms that combined make up an illness called either major depression or bipolar disorder. Your loved one may not have a clear understanding that his or her troubles are an illness. He may not be able to see the connection between what he is feeling and depression or mania. He might believe it's "just me" and that it's not responsive to any type of treatment.

He may lack insight into his illness—that special sense of self-awareness and perspective—and not grasp the cause of his deep despair or how to manage his symptoms. It may lead to day-to-day struggles as you try to help. Lack of insight may get in the way and become an obstacle to accepting his current experience as an illness and his ability to accept professional treatment, stick with recommended treatment, or accept any help from you.

Unrealistic expectations. The course of treatment for a mood disorder is often quite long compared to the treatment for other medical conditions. Seeing a response to talk therapy can take several months. Antidepressant medications are usually trial and error, and may take six to eight weeks before you begin to see any signs of improvement in the person. This requires extraordinary patience, yet many who have a mood disorder come to expect a "quick fix" or "magic pill" similar to when they receive a course of antibiotics for a strep throat infection. This is not a fair comparison. Also, some are not prepared to do the hard work of talk therapy. It is unrealistic to expect improvement in symptoms without some effort by the affected person. Engaging in psychotherapy and taking the steps to get better are indeed hard work, requiring active participation by your loved one. You can help by learning about mood disorders and treatment and by setting up realistic ideas for your loved one regarding what he can expect from treatment—a welcome improvement over the continued misery he would experience without treatment.

Turning down help. With depression or bipolar disorder, it may not be as simple as asking your family member or friend, "How can I help?" and then receiving feedback on what you can do. You may instead hear: "Leave me alone." "I just want to stay in bed." "You don't understand." "There's nothing anyone can do to help." Unlike other illnesses, someone who has a mood disorder may reject help rather than welcome it. This is because depression affects a person's mind and thinking.

Your friend or family member may be unable to cope using her regular methods she has always had to deal with other illnesses or stress. She may feel far beyond any hope or help, convinced that this is a permanent state that will never improve. She might believe that, even if she were to get better, she has nothing to offer anyone and will never have a life worth living, a meaningful career, or a fulfilling relationship. She could feel fundamentally flawed and defective, unlovable, and incompetent. Even if she has successfully overcome depression before, it's not uncommon for her to forget ever having felt well and so now denies it.

> When you're fatigued, it's sometimes easy to believe in the stigma that surrounds mental illness.

In depression, it's hard for the affected person to separate the illness symptoms from "just me." She may believe that her current state is her normal, usual self and forget what she was like before this depression episode. She may not recall that she ever had a sense of humor or was good at making friends. If your family member has bipolar disorder and is in a manic state, she may also lose *insight* and deny that she has an illness at all. She may angrily reject help, believing you're the one with the problem and who is misguided and narrow minded. This makes your job even more difficult.

Stigma and misunderstanding. Symptoms of depression often overlap with normal feelings such as sadness or fatigue, making it more difficult for you to know what's really going on. We now know that depression is a biologic medical condition. Even so, it's not unusual for people to wonder whether their family member or friend who has depression really has an illness. They may believe he is just lazy or lacks ambition. You might sometimes feel that your family member or friend is simply not trying hard enough to get better. Perhaps you think he could just "snap out of it" if he really wanted to. This can happen even if you are knowledgeable about depression and have only the best intentions.

I encourage you to let go of your guilt about having these thoughts on occasion, especially in private moments when you are tired and stressed. It's easy to understand depression as an illness when you're distanced from it. It is much more difficult to keep that in mind when you're living with someone day to day who has depression. Just try to be aware of these thoughts and recognize that such thoughts are not helpful and only contribute to the stress of caring for your family member.

Be aware, too, that mistaken beliefs about depression often complicate treatment. Most of us would encourage someone to take prescribed medications for diabetes, high blood pressure, or bronchitis. However, it's not uncommon for some of us to question whether treatments for depression are really necessary, whether they are a crutch or a Band-Aid, or perhaps even addictive. Even if you realize the errors in these statements, you know that others may wonder whether your family member "really needs to be taking those drugs." They may even urge him to stop taking them, against all medical advice. Gaining the support of these family members and friends can be difficult. This makes it harder for you and for your family member to stick with the recommended treatment.

Confidentiality and sharing information. Current federal regulations address the privacy of health information. These regulations are stricter for mental health disorders than for other medical conditions. This means that, if your family member is over age 18, her doctors or counselors are not allowed to share information with you without her explicit permission. This applies even if she is hospitalized in a psychiatric unit. As a result, you may feel shut out from her evaluation and treatment. You may also wonder whether the treatment team thinks you caused or contributed to your family member's depression. However, in an emergency, you can speak with her doctors. You can contribute valuable information about her, particularly when she can't communicate clearly herself. The treatment provider can receive this information without violating her privacy concerns. Mental health professionals will welcome your support and the perspective you provide as an ally in treatment.

> **Confidentiality rules can make you feel left out of your loved one's care and experience.**

Uncertain outcome. Although the treatment and outcome for medical problems such as a knee replacement or strep throat varies, there are still reliable guidelines and expectations for these conditions. Doctors can usually provide helpful guidance about the recovery time in days, weeks, or months. If you are helping a family member through one of these conditions, you can usually know what to expect and be able to plan your life around it. However, this is much more difficult to do with depression or bipolar disorder. Some people respond to the first treatment and are back to their old selves in a few months. Others don't respond as readily and have a more complicated treatment course. They may need to try many different medications and treatments. Their diagnosis may need refining over time, as more information becomes available. This can become a long, unpredictable journey. It's wise to attend to your own health and well-being in order to be able to support your family member during his recovery.

Lack of established routines. We usually know how to respond when a friend or family member has a serious medical problem like cancer, a heart attack, or other medical problem. We know when to call 9-1-1. We organize rides to appointments, accompany her to chemotherapy, and sit with her for hours as she recovers from its side effects. We bring casseroles and funny movies and organize fundraising walks. In contrast, we're not yet comfortable in knowing just what to do for a person who has depression or bipolar disorder. I wrote this book because I realized how you, as a well-meaning friend or family member, can spring into action when you are familiar with the diagnosis and how to help but often withdraw and don't know just what to do when it's a mood disorder.

There may be other challenges in caring for your loved one that you come across. I encourage you to step back and deal with each situation as it arises in a calm, neutral manner. Try to understand that your family member's or friend's thoughts and actions are driven by the illness and are not intentional. This will make it easier for you to deal with your own uncomfortable emotions.

The following story about Mike shows us how mood disorders can have a big impact on the family, those like you who are earnestly concerned while at the same time affected. In this example, when the individual keeps rejecting attempts to help him, friends and families become frustrated and feel powerless. It may take some creative thinking, and tough love, to get your family member the professional help he so badly needs.

Mike is a 48-year-old man who's worked as a car salesman for the past ten years, after being laid off from his job at an insurance company. He has always felt like a failure after that happened. He lives with his wife, Amy, and two teenage children in a small town. Lately, Mike has been moody and irritable, picking fights with his wife, and drinking a six-pack of beer each night after work. His sleep is fragmented, and he says he has no energy, so he stopped his jogging routine and has lost interest in other hobbies. He won't discuss any plans for their family with her, such as what to do for Thanksgiving. And he has become forgetful, neglecting chores around the house or promises he's made to others. Amy feels frustrated, which has led to a strain in their marriage. When asked by his wife about these changes and how he is feeling, he says, "Nothing's wrong! Get off my back!" and "Stop nagging me!" Mike seems to angrily reject all efforts by his wife and best friend, Joe, to help him, to support him, and to find out what's bothering him. "There's nothing anyone can do," he says. Then he closes himself off in their basement den, drinking all night. He refuses to go with her to the kids' soccer games on the weekends or out to dinner with friends. Amy wonders if he has depression, something she read about in a woman's magazine, and has tried to get him to see his family doctor— without success. She feels as though her hands are tied, that she can't force him to talk about it or to seek professional help, and that his new behaviors are disruptive to family life. The children wonder if he is angry with them or doesn't care for them anymore.

Amy is planning a family meeting to include Mike, his brother and sister-in-law, and his best friend, Joe. They plan to sit down with Mike and, without ganging up on him, describe what is different about him recently and raise their concerns. They hope that, in doing this, he will then gain some insight and agree to see his primary care physician for evaluation and referral to a mental health specialist.

Support and Communication Strategies

In this book, I walk you through some helpful things that you as a family member, significant other, or close friend can do for someone who is depressed. You will see that, often, it's a matter of knowing just what to say or do in the moment. This is easier said than done. So how do you know the most useful actions to take or words to say? First, remember that you—the family members and close friends—are the ones who provide daily support and encouragement, a very important element. You might then wonder what that support really involves. On an emotional level, "support . . . involves time spent listening, hearing and acknowledging the emotions that the patient is experiencing, and also advocating on the patient's behalf" (Buckman 1992, 67).

PROVIDING SUPPORT

Providing support is a good place to start. Although you may not realize it, supporting someone who is ill is usually a huge job. It's an effort that can continue 24 hours a day. It may at times be difficult and result in your own burnout. Take good care of yourself during this time so you remain better energized to care for your family member or friend. Chapter 17 can help you with this.

The overall goal in providing emotional support is for your family member or friend to know that you are listening and interested in what he thinks. This is an important message to get across to him. How do you best do this? Others in your situation find the following approach helpful. Focus your efforts on

- listening without judging
- hearing what he says
- responding with empathy to his words

An *empathic response* means that you try to identify with and understand your friend or family member's feelings or problems. Put yourself in his shoes. One of the most common challenges you may find is a breakdown in listening. (The causes are listed in table 7.1.) The rest of this chapter will offer effective listening and communication strategies.

You can provide other types of support as well, such as financial, physical, or household support. Everyone who experiences depression has different needs, and caregivers have different abilities to assist in these areas. Each type of support you offer may be appropriate at the time, depending on your family member or friend's age, personal circumstances, and extent of illness. You may offer to accompany your elderly parent to a doctor's appointment, help a friend with grocery shopping, or take your cousin's dog to the vet. Your goal is to help without making your family member or friend feel entirely dependent. It's important that you

- be clear and consistent in what you can and cannot offer in support
- set clear limits and expectations for both you and your family member or friend
- try not to promise anything you cannot deliver

COMMUNICATION STRATEGIES

Your family member or friend may feel helped now if he knows you are consistently there for him. This means you try to regularly set aside a time and place for private conversation to check in on how he is doing. Do you feel awkward doing this? That's not uncommon—many people in your position do. But most people who have depression actually find it helps to talk about it. Talking about it does not make the depression worse; your family member may be relieved to know that his depression symptoms make sense, that his symptoms have a name, and that his condition is common and legitimate. Try to show respect, dignity, and regard for his privacy in your words and actions. Make your best effort to accept what he says. Don't repeat anything he says in confidence.

Here's a suggestion for what you can do now: sit down with your family member or friend and encourage him to speak openly in his own words. Let him express his feelings and emotions without interruption. This will show him that his feelings and experiences are valid and important. You don't have to agree with what he says. Also, be especially careful not to appear judgmental or dismissive. Try to understand that someone who has depression is not always able or willing to talk about his feelings or what he privately discussed in therapy. You might feel shut out, but don't take it personally.

In this conversation, show that you are listening and have *heard* what he said. As you will learn, listening and hearing are two different skills. The following steps may help guide you in having a satisfactory dialogue with your loved one (Buckman, 1992):

> Keep everything in confidence unless it is a threat to his life and safety or that of others.

Prepare. Use open body language, which means making your best effort to do as many of the following as you can: sit down; remain calm; relax your posture without folding your arms, pointing your finger, or fidgeting; turn your body toward your family member or friend; give him your full attention and shut off your cell phone; make eye contact; and use a clear, calm voice.

Use active listening. This way of communicating tells him you are fully present and paying attention to what he is saying. It's not easy to do, especially if your mind tends to wander. If that happens, try to bring it right back to the topic. It gets easier to do with practice. Active listening is important to try because it often helps you to build rapport, understanding, and trust. It can help you avoid misunderstandings and frequently enables your family member or friend to open up. Here's how to use active listening:

- Focus on his words without allowing your mind to stray.
- Use open body language to show you are listening and interested.
- Make direct eye contact.
- Let him speak without interruption.
- Encourage him to talk by nodding your head and saying, "Tell me more" or "Um-hmm."
- Respond periodically by restating, reflecting, or summarizing his words.
- Ask open questions to draw him out, such as, "How did that make you feel?" "What do you think would happen if . . . ?"
- Tolerate short periods of silence. This can be difficult. He may be silent if his feelings are very intense or if he's deep in thought. Accept that for the moment. A short period of silence often gives him permission to feel or express his emotions. Occasionally, break the silence by asking, "What were you thinking of just now?"

Show that you have heard him: this indicates that you understand what he has said and that his words have meaning. In this way, you may be able to validate his feelings. You don't have to agree with him. Try to respond to him in one of the following ways:

- Repeat his exact words (repetition).
- Repeat what he says in your own words (paraphrase).
- Identify and state the emotion his words suggest (reflection).

Reflection effectively shows you have both heard and then interpreted what he said. If he says, "Life is no good. It's never going to change for me," you might respond with, "I hear that life feels no good to you right now and seems hopeless." This acknowledges his feelings and sense of hopelessness. Interpret his words as accurately as possible. Otherwise, you might lose the trust you've just worked to build. If you are unsure about the emotion he is feeling, avoid using the reflection response.

You can also show that you have heard your family member or friend by periodically summarizing what he says. This allows you to clarify what was said and lets him expand further on his thoughts. For example, you might say:

It appears that _____.
It sounds like _____.
What you seem to be saying is _____.
Is that the case? Do I understand correctly? _____.

Ask questions. Questions are a great way to show interest and to clarify facts so that you understand the point your family member or friend is trying to make. You can ask different types of questions in conversation; each may have a different impact on someone in distress. Some examples include:

- Closed question. A *closed question* is designed to obtain a specific answer. It allows only a few potential responses such as yes or no. It doesn't give your family member or friend a chance to express his feelings and emotions or describe a stressful situation. An example of a closed question is, "Did your doctor renew your prescription today?" (yes or no). Try to use this type of question sparingly.
- Open question. An *open question* allows your family member or friend to respond in any way he chooses. It gives him permission to talk openly about his feelings or experiences. Examples of an open question would be, "How did that make you feel?" "What did you make of that?" Try to use open questions often to learn more about what your family member may be feeling and why.

Respond. You may find several good ways of responding to your family member or friend in the course of a conversation. You can make a non-judgmental statement (repeat, paraphrase, or reflect), use body language such as a head nod, ask an open question, or be silent for a short period. Of these, the most effective response is often an empathic response, a type of reflection.

How do you provide an empathic response? To begin, try to identify the emotion your family member or friend may be feeling, such as sadness, anxiety, or fear. Then, think about where that emotion came from, such as from a previous experience he had. Next, do your best to put them both together and respond in a way that shows you understand the connection between the two. For example, if he is upset about not being able to participate on the track team because of his illness, you might say, "You sound really sad about missing the track season this year and not being able to compete with your team because of your depression." This shows him that you both hear and understand his distress. In this way, you have identified his emotion (sad) and where it came from (missing the track season) and why (because of his depression).

> An empathic response is often the most effective response.

Or, in another example, if she is distraught and says that nobody likes her, your most effective response could be to say, "It must be really awful to feel unlovable when your friends don't call." You have identified her emotion (awful and unlovable) and its source (because her friends don't call). A word of caution. Use this technique only if you really think you know what your loved one is feeling—don't guess, as that often backfires.

Listening is considered an art. As you practice, you generally improve at it. This is true for most people. Be aware of the ways we all can unconsciously block effective listening and make your best effort to avoid them. Blocks to effective listening include making assumptions without knowing the facts, mind reading what the other person is thinking, making judgments, filtering out pieces of information (avoiding hearing some of the details), or daydreaming. Blocks to effective listening are described in table 7.1.

The value of good communication skills is demonstrated in this next story about Maya and Jeff. In it we can see how she learns effective listening and supportive techniques as a concerned family member, and the impact that has on his depression. These skills do not come naturally or easy to most of us and take some practice to get good at it. In the long run, your loved one who has depression will appreciate your effort.

TABLE 7.1. **Blocks to Effective Listening**
• Making assumptions (without the facts)
• Mind reading (when you conclude you know what someone is thinking without the facts)
• Filtering out what he's saying (e.g., when you avoid hearing some of the details)
• Judging what someone is saying
• Changing the subject to yourself or another topic
• Comparing his experience to someone else's
• Identifying (when you refer to your own similar experience)
• Rehearsing (when you focus on what you're going to say next)
• Daydreaming or not paying attention
• Giving advice
• Sparring, put-downs, sarcasm, or debating a point
• Needing to be right at any cost
• Placating the person

Maya is a 39-year-old woman whose husband Jeff is being treated for major depression. At first, she did not know how to respond to the situation, what to say or do. So, she went for a visit to her primary care physician and received some practical advice on being a supportive spouse. Maya began by making an effort to be there and really listen *to Jeff, without distractions, whenever he was willing to talk. It was hard to keep her mind from drifting to other topics and to stay focused on what he was saying even when she disagreed with the specific content of his words. Her primary care physician said to think about these wandering thoughts like a stray leaf that falls on the windshield of her car on a foggy day, with the windshield wipers slowly brushing it away. That seemed to help.*

Next, she tried to accept that what Jeff said and felt was valid for him and that she should not be judgmental or say things that dismissed his feelings like, "Oh, that's ridiculous!" That was also hard to do. It took a lot to curb her tongue, to not respond abruptly to his comments. Maya made an effort to acknowledge Jeff's thoughts, feelings, and emotions as legitimate, even if she sensed they were not accurate, and to reflect on his words by saying, "It sound like you're saying . . ." She read about using empathy—putting yourself in the other person's shoes to try to understand how he feels—and she tried that approach. She learned about taking deep breaths to stay calm when sticky or difficult subjects arose, how to make eye contact, and how to position your body to indicate you are interested and listening.

To let him know she fully heard him, Maya tried to remain focused on the conversation; to nod her head in understanding; to offer supportive comments, such as "I'm so sorry you have to deal with this illness"; and to ask thoughtful open-ended questions, such as "How did that make you feel?" All of this was new to her and took practice. She did not get it right away, but eventually Maya became a pretty good supportive listener.

Jeff responded positively to Maya's efforts. He felt more supported and less alone, that someone in this world cared enough and understood his issues. He was able to open up to Maya at times, which was unusual for a person like him who was raised to be a strong, macho-type man, hiding his innermost thoughts and feelings. This style of communication also strengthened their relationship.

If your loved one becomes upset, his or her ability to think and reason declines. This can happen for a lot of reasons and is not uncommon. At these moments, he is not able to address his thoughts or problems in a clear and logical manner. It is useless for you or others to argue with him. It's best to step back and allow him some time to cool off, and then make yourself available to talk when he is ready. Try not to express you own anger or frustration with him. If you do become angry and frustrated, this is a sign that you may be fatigued and overwhelmed by the situation. This is a good time for you to take a break as well. Many people in your position have found support groups for families to be helpful.

> **Stay calm if your loved one appears angry and hostile.**

If your friend or family member appears angry or hostile during your conversation, it's generally not helpful to respond in a similar angry manner. That can often escalate the situation. It may also add to your own personal stress. Instead, try to stay calm, step back, and show that you recognize the source of his anger and emotions. Again, do this only if you think you understand the source of his anger—don't guess here. Making incorrect assumptions about his thoughts or feelings may only fuel his anger. If you think you know, you might say, "It must make you feel angry to lose a position on your team this year." This identifies his emotion, lets him know you understand his loss, and allows him the opportunity to respond.

Many things can cause your family member or friend to feel angry when he is ill with any prolonged medical problem, including an episode of depression. (Examples of anger and its causes are presented in table 7.2.) He could be angry with his personal situation and having his life turned upside down by depression. He might be trying to cope with changes—in his daily routine away from work, school, friends, or colleagues; in his financial status; or in his recreational opportunities. He could be upset at having to deal with a mental illness or angry with himself, his health care providers, you because you are there, a family member who doesn't understand his struggles, or an employer for letting him go. Also, realize that during depression episodes some people, such as adult men or adolescents, may react more readily with irritability and anger instead of a low mood.

Keep in mind the following important point: wait until your family member's concerns have been stated and heard before you offer any reassuring words (such as "Things always work out"). If you do so too early, he might perceive it as a brush-off and may feel that his concerns are not valid.

TABLE 7.2. Anger in Your Family Member or Friend

Your family member or friend may feel angry with himself, you, others, or outside forces. He may believe any or all have negatively influenced him or his illness. The source may be inappropriate, and he may have no basis for such hostility. It may not seem rational to you as an observer. It is important, however, to understand what is behind his fury. Here is a list of potential targets for his anger:

Anger against the illness

He may feel anger at his symptoms, being disabled by the illness, the loss of freedom to do as he pleases, or the unfairness of it all (why me?).

Anger against his loss of control and lack of power

He may be angry because of his inability to control his life. He may feel overly dependent on friends, family, and his medical team.

Anger against his perceived loss of potential

He may feel anger because he believes his future hopes and dreams are lost.

Anger against himself

He may be angry with himself if he believes he caused his own illness. He may feel betrayed by his body and angry at his own negative attitude.

Anger against friends and family

He may resent the fact that friends and family enjoy good health. He may still be angry as a result of old family arguments. He may hate receiving advice, charity, and sympathy from others. He may believe that friends or family contributed to his illness, whether appropriate or inappropriate. He may feel angry and abandoned when he feels others are withdrawing from him.

Anger against medical and other health professional teams

He may blame his health care team for any news regarding his diagnosis, treatment, and outcome. He may feel he's given up control to his doctors or resent the perceived good health of his medical team. He may feel angry if he believes his mental health providers are cold, insensitive, or do not listen. He may be angry if there are communication gaps, if he is not part of the decision-making process, or if he does not agree with their decisions.

Anger against "outside forces"

He may be angry with his workplace situation (whether appropriately or inappropriately) or angry with his daily environment at home.

Anger against God

He may feel anger if he thinks that God or the divine has abandoned him. He may believe that God is unjustly punishing him. He may think that after all his years of keeping faith and religious observances, he is seeing a poor return on his efforts.

Source: Adapted from Robert Buckman, *How to Break Bad News: A Guide for Health Care Professionals* (Johns Hopkins University Press, 1992), 138–139.

8

Helpful Approaches

HELPFUL APPROACHES

As you approach your family member or friend who has depression, keep in mind that the suggestions in this chapter have helped many people just like you and her. They are offered in addition to the communication and support strategies that were described in chapter 7. Because following these suggestions may involve changing how you interact with someone, you might consider trying these approaches one at a time before adding a second and then a third. You will see they often make a difference.

For more information on the topics in this chapter, I recommend the website Families for Depression Awareness at familyaware.org. This is a wonderful organization for families, and the website is rich with useful material in educational webinars, video, and print.

Treat Your Loved One Normally

Do your best to treat your family member normally, which means making an effort to include her in your usual everyday activities and family and social plans. Make it clear that you expect her to participate in pleasurable activities as well as to share in the daily chores around the house and keep up with responsibilities at school or work. She does not want to feel left out or different because of her illness. Let her be the one to determine whether it's too much to handle. Help her modify her activities as needed, but try not to give her an easy out.

If she needs to take a leave of absence from work or school, do your best to treat it as a temporary setback, not a failure. You can expect her to slowly get back on track as her depression lifts. Many people with depression find their moods slowly lift as they make contact with others. This isn't always the case, however. Some people end up feeling worse after they see friends or family doing well and enjoying their lives, making a comparison to their own current misery.

Set Limits as Needed

You may need to set limits on your family member's or friend's daily behavior. This may be difficult for both of you. Try to see that he understands you expect him to abide by the rules of the household or social group. You might even have to encourage him to bathe, wash his hair, and wear clean clothes. Since it's important that a person who has depression not isolate himself from others, try to get him to share dinner each night with the family or social group.

Set Behavior Expectations

You may also need to set expectations on how she relates with other family members or friends. Depression or bipolar disorder does not give anyone the right to be overly argumentative or demanding of others' time and patience. Try to let her know you expect her to act calmly, with courtesy and good manners toward other family members and friends, no matter how down, irritable, or bad she feels. You may need to specify boundaries on specific behaviors, curfews, and the use of alcohol and street drugs. If your family member begins to indulge in late-night drinking binges, you will want

> Mood disorders are not an excuse for abusive behavior.

to let her know that this is not healthy or acceptable in the household. You may need to both clearly agree on what time she is expected home every evening and how she spends her free time. This is particularly important for young adults and adolescents. Try to make your expectations clear and stick to them. This can be a source of conflict in some families. If she resists or rebels, your best strategy may be to remain firm. Try to avoid giving in just because of her illness.

Try to Provide Hope

> *There is no medicine like hope, no incentive so great and no tonic*
> *so powerful as the expectation of something better tomorrow.*
> —ORISON SWETT MARDEN, FOUNDER, *SUCCESS* MAGAZINE

Often in depression, a person loses hope for herself, her future, and her world. It can be incapacitating. Your words and example can indicate that you have not lost hope for her—that you have expectations for her future and believe things will improve. This can be a powerful message. How do you convey it?

One way is to try to keep her plans for the future alive in conversation, even if those plans have to be modified for now. If she has to take a leave of absence from work or school, you could say, "I expect that next fall when

you get back to work [school, team, or committee] you'll be able to _____."
She may feel encouraged on hearing that you expect she will successfully
return to her usual activities. Your goal is to treat displaced plans as temporary setbacks, not failures.

If she lacks hope or optimism, try to suggest she "borrow" hope from
someone who cares for her and believes she has potential. That person could
be you. You might say, "I sense that you don't feel hopeful about _____ right
now, but I do. Why don't you let me keep hope alive for you?" Through your
eyes she may begin to see the possibilities in her life return. It may be difficult for you to maintain a positive, upbeat attitude when you too are struggling and all else seems grim. Try to focus on the fact that this is a treatable
biological illness with ups and downs.

Set Realistic Expectations

Next, do your best to set realistic expectations for your family member or
friend. Convey to him that *right now* he may not be able to do everything
he used to do—and that's okay. Right now he may have to modify his plans
and responsibilities. This is related to the depression and improves for most
people. Your family member may feel validated knowing you don't believe
he's weak or a failure or that he's lazy or faking it. Try to accept what he can
do now and encourage him to stretch his wings as he is able. You might
gently suggest he get involved in a hobby or an activity he once enjoyed,
return to work or school part time, or perhaps volunteer, at a pace he can
handle now.

Volunteering is of tremendous value in restoring confidence after the
isolation of depression. It provides a great transition, a sense of purpose
and gets your loved one back into being sociable and in a different mindset.
When he or she volunteers, he has to present himself in a pleasant manner,
interact and connect with other people, and become accountable to others.
I've learned that you get back much more in volunteering than you give.

It's sometimes a challenge to keep realistic expectations for your family
member in what he or she might be able to do now, and not convey a bit of
your own personal disappointment. Focusing on the *now* is not to say that
those things he used to do are never going to be attainable; rather, they just
need to be approached in small, realistic steps *at the moment*. Your son does
not have to pursue a full semester of hard-core academics or a position on
the soccer team right now; he can take the semester off or schedule a lighter
course load for the next few months until his symptoms improve. This is
okay and will not diminish him as a person or impact his overall life. This is
a temporary setback; as he recovers, so will his interest and drive.

Show Realistic Optimism

It can be particularly helpful to show realistic optimism. *Realistic optimism* is a reasonable view of the future that involves hope and the confidence that, with enough hard work and determination, things will turn out well. It means discussing his realistic plans for the future and supporting his efforts to get there. Some people take their illness as an opportunity to rethink their ambitions and life direction and may make other more appealing decisions about their life goals and aspirations.

If your family member or friend has had more than one episode of depression in his life, try not to assume he will automatically know how to handle the next one. This isn't realistic. It often takes a lot of time, effort, and skill working with a mental health professional for someone who has depression to successfully manage his illness. It may require a great deal of insight and practice on his part to anticipate the triggers; handle the difficult times of life, such as dreaded holidays or certain relationships, and take the steps to minimize their effects. This can be frustrating to you as an observer. Patience and understanding are essential.

NEGATIVE THOUGHTS AND DISTORTED THINKING

In all of us there is a close connection between our thoughts, feelings, and behaviors. It's common for those who experience depression to see themselves, their experiences, their future, and the world through a distorted, negative lens they strongly believe is accurate. The depressed mind tends to make errors in thinking, interpreting and twisting an event in different ways. This happens automatically, not on purpose. It means that many things your loved one sees, thinks, and believes will automatically have a negative twist or bias to it and may cause *automatic negative thoughts*, which can often be a source of distress to the person. Automatic negative thoughts are extreme and spontaneous distortions in thinking; in the moment, your loved one may strongly believe that these thoughts are true. Common negative thoughts include, "I'm a loser," "I can't do anything right," "Nobody likes me," "Everybody hates me," or "I always drop the ball."

Dealing with twisted and negative thoughts is the foundation of cognitive behavioral therapy (CBT), a kind of talk therapy (psychotherapy) used successfully in those who have depression and bipolar disorder. In CBT, your loved one learns to identify and change distorted thinking patterns, inaccurate beliefs, and unhelpful behaviors. CBT is a way to help her look at her thoughts and determine when she is thinking in a rational or an irrational way. Your family member learns to monitor, to challenge, and to replace her distorted or negative thoughts with more realistic ones and to recognize the connection between her thoughts, feelings, and behaviors.

> *Automatic negative thoughts are extreme and spontaneous distortions in thinking that overwhelm a person's reasoning.*

Addressing the many different types of twisted or distorted thinking, such as those that follow, is fundamental to CBT. These thoughts are usually repetitive, not necessarily logical or based on fact, and can seem frustrating from your point of view. You don't have to fully understand or remember the different types of thought distortions in this list. Just know that they are possibilities and that someone who has depression may unintentionally and spontaneously think this way.

Different Types of Distorted Thinking

The following are examples of how a person can unintentionally twist or distort her thinking.

Filtering. A person puts his entire focus on the negative aspects of a situation, ignoring (filtering out) the positive. He might reject or minimize his good qualities or experiences and insist they "don't count." An otherwise average-looking or attractive person might think, "I have a zit on my nose; now I'm really ugly and everyone will think I'm a freak!"

Polarized thinking. A person thinks in extremes: good or bad, black or white, all or none. He sees nothing in-between. A worst extreme is when someone cooks a meal that isn't perfect and sees himself as a "total failure."

Jumping to conclusions. A person negatively interprets what will happen in life without having any facts. There are different ways this can occur:

- *Predicting how someone else is going to think or react.* A person might conclude that she knows what others are feeling or thinking or why they act a certain way without their saying so. She might think, "Everybody is going to be laughing at me" without having any reason or basis for coming to that conclusion.
- *Predicting what is going to happen in the future.* A person might be convinced he knows that things will turn out badly but has no supporting evidence for thinking that way. He might think, "I know I'm not going to be able to do this project right, and I'll get fired from my job."

Overgeneralizing. A person comes to an overall conclusion based on one single event or piece of evidence. He sees a single event as permanent and expects it to occur over and over again, often using the words "always" or "never." A person might think, "My date didn't call me back, and I know I'll never get another date with anyone else ever again."

Global labeling. An extreme form of overgeneralization in which a person combines one or two negative qualities into a negative judgment and applies a label to herself or others. A person might label himself a "loser" based on one less-than-perfect thing he said or did. She might also blame a problem in her marriage on her "jerk husband" and assume no responsibility for it.

Expecting the worst. A person magnifies things out of proportion and expects the worst outcome, a disaster; he exaggerates his own negatives (errors) or somebody else's positives (achievements). Following a minor incident at work, a person might think, "I lost a client at work, and now everyone will think I'm totally stupid and nobody will ever be friends with me."

Discounting the positive. A person minimizes his own positive qualities or experiences, insisting they don't count. "I only passed the test because the teacher made it so easy. Anybody could do it."

Personalizing. A person thinks that everything other people say or do is a reaction to him personally. Or he assumes responsibility for outside events and blames himself for an event outside of his control. Someone on a sports team might think, "I dropped the ball, and we lost the entire game because of me" when in fact it was the whole team who was responsible for the loss.

Reward fallacy. A person expects that all of his sacrifices and self-denial will pay off, and he feels bitter and resentful when it doesn't happen.

Emotions rule. A person believes that what she feels must automatically be true, that her negative emotions are the true and accurate state. A person might think,"I feel so stupid, so I *must* be stupid. It must be true."

For more on this topic, I refer the reader to *Feeling Good: The New Mood Therapy* (Burns 2009).

What Can You Do?

You may help your family member or friend greatly by gently encouraging her to challenge the negative thought distortions she may have. Although some family members fear that talking about it may make things worse, that's not usually the case. You can try this now using one or more of the following suggestions. They are not meant for you to act as her therapist. She may or may not be willing or able to discuss these issues with you on any given day.

- Help her replace automatic negative thoughts with alternative, more realistic thoughts. If she says, "Nobody likes me. I have no friends," you might gently ask her to really think about that thought and where it comes from. Suggest she replace it with something accurately reflecting her life today. You might say, "I hear you feel like you are unlovable and have no friends. That must feel awful. What about the people in your book club? Didn't you tell me some of them like you?" Let her be the one to come up with the alternative thought: "Well, I do have a few friends in my book club." Then ask, "Where do you think that thought comes from?" See if she feels better after this exercise. Often, this is the case.

When a negative thought, belief, or interpretation of an event causes your loved one distress, it's helpful to examine the evidence for and against it. This will help her identify and change thoughts that are based on inaccurate assumptions. You could start by having her focus on one particular negative thought. She will need a piece of paper with three columns, one for stating the problem thought or belief, one titled "Evidence FOR" the thought and one titled "Evidence AGAINST" the thought. Have her consider the evidence in her life *against* the negative thought and the evidence *for* the negative thought and fill in the two columns. See the example in table 8.1. If she has trouble doing this exercise, she may need to ask friends or family for suggestions. Many people who have depression find more evidence against the negative thought than for it. Seeing a visual image in this way, your family member or friend may realize the error of her thinking. It may help to lift her mood.

Remind her that the negative feeling and emotions she now experiences and perceives to be true are actually temporary events inside her mind and not *facts*. Thoughts are not facts. Feelings are not facts. Have your loved one gather evidence as to the truth of something that she is bothered by and perceives to be real. It is usually hard for a person to dispute evidence in front of her. Have her focus on the facts.

• Try to help her challenge negative thoughts by asking your family member or friend to remember her past successes. If she believes she's a failure, as many people who have depression do, she will probably deny ever having any past successful outcomes. The negative thoughts in depression often cause a person to believe she has failed in life, is incompetent, or is a loser. Point out her achievements, whether in school, at work, in sports, or with a hobby. You might ask, "What about the time you were recognized at work for your project?" or "Remember the time you won a blue ribbon in the 5 K road race?" With real-life evidence before her, denial becomes more difficult.

TABLE 8.1. Evidence For and Against		

When a thought, a belief, or an interpretation of an event causes you distress, it's helpful to examine the evidence for and against it. This will help you identify and change thoughts based on inaccurate assumptions.

Step 1. Identify a negative or distressing thought.

Step 2. Gather evidence for and against that thought.

• Collect specific evidence about the thought to check its accuracy.

• Ask others who know you well for their realistic, honest feedback about the thought.

• Seek out experiences that counteract your negative beliefs. For example, go out, do an activity, and observe what really happens. You will see firsthand the evidence against them.

Step 3. Look at your list realistically and see where the evidence lies.
Ask yourself: Is your belief inherently true, or is it an internalized message from your environment? If you find it is true, think about what is in your power to change.

BELIEF OR THOUGHT	EVIDENCE FOR . . .	EVIDENCE AGAINST . . .

Source: Susan J. Noonan, *Managing Your Depression: What You Can Do to Feel Better* (Johns Hopkins University Press, 2013), 99–100.

She may push aside those negative beliefs and accept some degree of competence in herself.

- Ask your family member or friend how she successfully dealt with a tough situation in the past. She may initially deny ever having overcome an adversity. Try to use gentle persuasion to remind her of those events. You could say, "I remember the time you had a difficult project to do and you _____." or "What about the time when _____ happened and you were able to _____?" Recognizing these successes may boost her self-confidence and eventually her mood.

- Try to get your family member or friend to explore what's behind her negative thoughts. Where and when did they start? Ask her whether the issues underlying these thoughts are current and bother her now or if they are from years past. You might ask, "Are you just now thinking about _____ [negative thought]? Did this come up recently, or have you been thinking about it for a while? How does it affect you now?" Past experiences can often haunt someone who has depression. Thinking about them constantly, called *rumination*, is both common and unhelpful. Ask her what's in her power to try to change now. Encourage her to put aside negative thoughts stemming from the past. This could bring her a great deal of relief.

STRENGTHS AND PERSONAL QUALITIES

Often in an episode of depression a person may lose sight of his or her personal strengths, traits, and achievements. She may quickly deny that she has any redeeming qualities at all, as her world is colored by a dark, negative lens.

Listing our strengths, weaknesses, and achievements can build self-esteem and protect against depression.

This contributes to a loss of self-esteem and self-confidence and fosters depression. It's hard to break this cycle.

Your role as a supportive friend or family member can be to assist her in realistically identifying her strengths (and weaknesses), positive traits, and accomplishments. Honestly state what you observe and admire in her. Once recognized and acknowledged, you can then help her build on them. Perhaps she has always had a good sense of humor, is a pretty good artist or baker, a loyal friend, completed a 5 K road race, or is skilled at computers. Gently remind her of these things on occasion as you encourage her to develop them further. Better yet, have her create her own list of her strengths and weaknesses, positive traits and characteristics, and personal achievements to have on hand.

Why is this important to do? For one, it becomes a powerful tool for her to recapture the essence of her underlying person and builds on her self-esteem. That can be protective against future episodes of depression. For more on how to do this and the process of defining your baseline, see my book *Take Control of Your Depression: Strategies to Help You Feel Better Now* (Noonan 2018).

WATCH FOR WARNING SIGNS OF DEPRESSION

Many people who experience depression or bipolar disorder exhibit warning signs that become obvious just before their depression or mania worsens. Warning signs are distinct changes from the person's usual thoughts, feelings, behaviors, actions, daily routines, or self-care habits. You may notice them right before a decline in mood. Warning signs can include:

- More negative thoughts
- More feelings of hopelessness, sadness, irritability, anxiety, or fatigue
- Appetite loss
- Sleep disruption
- Changes in personal hygiene, such as failure to bathe
- Difficulty with daily routines
- Loss of interest in previously enjoyed activities
- Excessive alcohol use
- Slipping grades in school

Each person has a characteristic, unique pattern of warning signs. Sometimes, these are subtle. Try to learn about and look for your family member's or friend's particular type and pattern of warning signs. If you notice any of them, that is the time to call for professional help and follow the Basics of Mental Health outlined in chapter 3. Recognizing her warning signs early may give you the chance to step in and try to change the course of her depression or bipolar episode. The following story of Jan and David shows the subtle warning signs of depression that you need to pay attention to.

> *Jan is just beside herself. She's been married to David for 15 years. Together, they have two children, ages 9 and 11. Jan works outside the home part time, and David works full time as a computer programmer, a job he enjoyed until the past few months. Since then he's been coming home from work irritable and solemn, reluctant to speak to Jan about any issues going on at work. This is unlike him. She doesn't know if anything*

happened, but she guesses David is upset about work-related budget con-straints, tight deadlines, and a boss who's been particularly critical lately. But she's not sure because David clams up and won't talk to her.

Instead, he takes it out on her and the kids, finding fault with the way she cooks, the kids' behavior, the house—just about anything. He has stopped jogging and working out, activities he always enjoyed, and refuses to take the children to their soccer games and birthday parties. His best friend and brother have called to speak with him a few times, and he won't take their calls. He says he's "too tired."

Several times, Jan has found David up in the middle of the night, unable to sleep, drinking a few beers (he says beer isn't really alcohol) or scotch. Lately, he's taken to having a scotch or two right when he gets home at night. One day Jan found a bottle of half-opened vodka hidden in his workroom. When she expressed her concerns and suggested he visit their family doctor, David snapped at her and told her to leave him alone.

Jan is concerned for their children and doesn't want them to see David's behavior or ride in the car with him. She is planning to remove all alcohol from the house. Jan is persistent and plans to get his brother and best friend to sit down with him. She hopes they can get him to open up and agree to see his doctor.

As you can see, David is showing the warning signs of depression. He's irritable and withdrawn, has trouble sleeping, is drinking to excess and has changed his usual routine. Jan has recognized this and has plans to inter-vene and encourage him to seek professional help.

SET BOUNDARIES

You may find that a person who has depression or bipolar disorder can occa-sionally be difficult to live with. Her behavior may distress you and others in your family or social group. She may be upset, irritable, or very sad. She may not think clearly and take her feelings out on you and others.

As this book makes clear, it's important to understand what depression is. However, use your understanding of the illness to cope, not to excuse unacceptable behavior. Family life will be easier and of higher quality if you set boundaries when needed. *Boundaries* are rules or limits on behavior that you and the person who has depression agree on. They provide a feeling of safety for your family member when things feel out of control. Work with her to set these boundaries in a firm but compassionate way.

Here's how you might go about doing it: Together, you both agree beforehand about what will be considered problematic or socially unacceptable behavior. This is generally not an easy conversation. Your family member may give you a hard time and be unwilling to go along. Your best approach is to be firm and consistent. You might begin by defining what behavior you will or will not tolerate. For example, you might specify limits on late-night activities, alcohol or illegal substance use, or failing to bathe. Try to be clear about what the con-

> Agree together on what is unacceptable behavior and the consequences of misbehavior.

sequences for misbehavior will be; follow through with them consistently if there is a breach. Here are some examples of boundaries you may want to include in your agreement (adapted from Sheffield 1998):

1. *Compliance with treatment and medication.* For any number of reasons, your family member may stop taking her psychiatric medications. These drugs can make her groggy or nauseated or have other side effects. She may worry that her friends or employer will judge her harshly if they know she takes medication.

People who have depression or bipolar disorder may get fed up with all of the talk therapy (psychotherapy) sessions they are required to attend in order to get better. Talking about life events and intimate feelings can be hard. It brings up strong emotions. Traveling to sessions, keeping track of schedules, filling out insurance paperwork, paying medical bills—all can lead someone to drop a session or two or decide to quit therapy entirely.

Stopping medications and talk therapy can interfere with recovery and well-being. A team approach is often most effective to help convince someone to continue treatment. It's most effective if you, other family members, and her health care provider work together to encourage her cooperation with her treatment plan. Try to find out what caused her to stop the medications and see whether you can help her solve that issue. Remind her that consistency with medications and treatment may often help her achieve the goals she so strongly desires. Use whatever means are available to get her to agree to the overall treatment plan.

2. *Unacceptable behavior.* Sometimes you must specify just what behaviors you will not tolerate in your household or family unit. This could be late nights, drinking or drugs, stealing, gambling, lack of self-care, skipping school, failure to contribute to household chores or joint responsibilities, or anything that disrupts the family. Be clear and firm on what will and will not be acceptable and remain consistent in the consequences for any breaches in your agreement.

3. *Verbal abuse.* A person who has depression or bipolar disorder may become so irritable and agitated that she feels and appears out of control. You may have to establish boundaries or rules against verbal outbursts of anger, insults, and verbal abuse toward you and other family members. Send her a clear message that you will not tolerate this kind of behavior. Setting boundaries may help her regain some control over her emotions. Deep down, she will thank you for it.

4. *Physical abuse.* Setting boundaries around physical abuse is a must. Never tolerate this type of behavior. Hitting, punching a wall, fist fighting, breaking objects, or other forms of violence may be your family member's way to express his frustration or anger. He does not know how else to express his emotions. That is not an excuse for bad behavior.

5. *Manipulation.* Some people who experience depression engage in subtle games of manipulation to get their own way. Your family member may attempt to look or sound helpless or incompetent so you or others will do things for her. Do not buy into this. Despite her depression and bipolar disorder, she may still be capable of doing many things for herself. Try not to do for her what she is capable of doing for herself. Set expectations with her about what you will and will not do.

Tough Love

Your family member's behavior may be so trying that you need to apply a tough love approach. Perhaps he is extremely argumentative, angry, abusive, or hurting himself, friends, or other family members. Use the tough love tactic to stay firm while loving.

Tough love is a method in which your troubled child or teen sees your love for him while you apply a firm and consistent approach in discipline, expectations, boundaries, and limits and follow through on the consequences of misbehavior as appropriate. In this model, your teen or young adult is considered responsible for his behavior, makes choices, and is held accountable for his (bad) choices. Remember that this approach is based on your love for your family member; you are acting in his best interest. You may need to remind him of your love and affection repeatedly.

> Try not to feel guilty for using a tough love approach. It requires strength on your part.

You might communicate that you will stop helping him with _____ until he clearly indicates he is willing to help himself. Or you might take privileges away from your rebellious teenager until he can show you he is able to comply with treatment and care for himself safely.

Zach's story in chapter 12 illustrates the difficulty in identifying the warning signs of depression in a teenager. You might not be sure if your family member is in a phase of adolescent behavior or if this is an indication of illness. This example shows that setting limits on daily behavior with a tough love approach, such as taking away the car keys until Zach can demonstrate he can care for himself, can be a useful and responsible step for parents to take.

MENTAL HEALTH FIRST AID

An additional set of helpful tools is called First Aid for Depression, a movement for families and friends that began in Australia in 2001. Mental Health First Aid is a national program in the United States and over 25 countries to teach the skills to respond to the signs of mental illness and substance abuse. It further describes the program as "the help provided to a person who has a mental health problem or is in a mental health crisis . . . given until appropriate professional treatment is received or the crisis resolves." The concept is to train family members, friends, and other responders to know what to look for and how to respond in an urgent mental health situation. It is similar in concept to CPR classes that train people to respond to someone in the midst of a medical emergency. Evidence behind the program shows that it effectively builds mental health literacy, or knowledge, and helps people identify, understand, and respond to signs of mental illness.

These intervention strategies are taught in eight-hour training programs originally created by Mental Health First Aid Australia, a national nonprofit charity focused on mental health training and research. The organization provides interesting and effective ways to respond to a person's depression. Guidelines are available at www.mhfa.com.au. In the United States, Mental Health First Aid USA can be found at www.mentalhealthfirstaid.org. Its goal is to provide free courses in prevention and early intervention. It is available to the general public. The course content teaches you a five-step action plan (ALGEE) with the skills to

- assess the risk of suicide or harm
- listen nonjudgmentally
- reassure and provide information
- encourage appropriate professional help
- foster self-help and other support strategies

Mental Health First Aid USA is administered by the National Center for Community Behavioral Healthcare, the Maryland State Department of Health and Mental Hygiene, and the Missouri Department of Mental Health.

9

What You Can Do Now

When you picked up this book, one of your questions might have been "How do I begin?" As you've read in previous chapters, the first thing to do is to be there, listen, and support your family member or friend who has depression. Self-help and self-care strategies are often useful, and your role is to encourage these efforts. This includes the Basics of Mental Health mentioned in chapter 3. Then try to focus on helping your loved one find professional treatment. After she's engaged in treatment, try to keep the Quick Tips for Caregivers (table 9.1) in mind:

TABLE 9.1. Quick Tips for Caregivers
Be there
Listen without judging
Use active listening, hearing, and respond with empathy
Provide support
Maintain hope
Keep realistic expectations for your family members
Help her confront negative thoughts
Do what you say you're going to do
Know the symptoms of depression or bipolar disorder. Learn about the illness
Know the warning signs of suicide. Call for help as needed
Encourage her to stick to the Basics of Mental Health
If you're a parent, you may need to set boundaries
Pace yourself
Emphasize that you're in this together—and mean it

It can take several weeks before a person who has depression sees a response to treatment. This is the most challenging time. Try to encourage your family member to be patient and stick with the proposed treatment plan.

This chapter provides you with some ideas to help your family member, organized by each of the main symptoms of depression. Keep in mind that she will most often experience a combination of symptoms at the same time, and that this combination will be different for each person. You may then have to overlap and customize your approach to her based on the suggestions that follow.

STEPS FOR ALTERED MOOD SYMPTOMS

If your family member shows persistent sadness or irritability, your initial response may be to listen and acknowledge this. You can do this by asking open questions and helping her explore her feelings without prying. You could begin with an observation such as "You seem to be very sad [or irritable] today." Some people open up and begin to talk at this point. If you get no response, you could go on to ask, "What do you think is the reason for this? Has anything happened?" Your family member may realize that her overall sadness is not related to any one thing in particular. Or she may find that something triggered her sadness, such as a major loss or disappointment. It may be one or several things.

After identifying the potential cause of her sadness or irritability, you might ask her to think of ways she can deal with it. Is there anything she can do to repair or replace the loss or change the impact it has on her? If so, try to help her find a solution. The following is often an effective strategy in *problem solving*:

1. Identify the problem.
2. Get accurate information about the problem.
3. Consider the options and alternative solutions.
4. Identify the necessary steps to address the problem.
5. Determine who she needs to assist her.

If she finds no concrete ways to change the facts, try to shift the focus of your conversation to coping with it.

What do I mean by coping? *Coping strategies* are the things we all do to ease the stressors and challenges of daily life. People use a wide range of tactics for this purpose. They include distraction, relaxation exercises, self-soothing strategies, mindfulness meditation, physical exercise, humor, and other techniques. You might begin by asking your family member what she has done in the past to successfully cope with similar sadness or loss. You could say, "What has helped you in the past when you have felt this way?" If she can identify a strategy or two, which might be something like physical exercise or humor, ask if she's able to engage in those coping skills now. You could say, "Would you like to go for a run now or watch something on Netflix?" This is often a helpful approach for people in similar situations. Examples of other effective coping strategies she might try include:

- *Distracting yourself from the problem.* Refocus attention on social activities, hobbies, physical exercise, sports, reading, puzzles, music, movies, or volunteering.
- *Relaxation techniques.* Herbert Benson ([1975] 2000) describes an easy one in *The Relaxation Response.* Begin by relaxing one muscle group in your body at a time. Slowly relax every other muscle group until all tension is released. Another technique, *mindfulness meditation*, is also easy to fit into your day (Kabat-Zinn 1994). In this practice, you stay present in the moment by paying attention, on purpose and nonjudgmentally, to what you are doing. You let go of worry about the past or future.
- *Mindfulness meditation.* Many people find it helpful to practice mindfulness meditation five minutes at a time, once or ideally twice a day. Here's how:
  - Sit in a comfortable chair.
  - Close your eyes.
  - Become aware of your breathing.
  - Focus on each breath.
  - Pay attention to the present moment: your breathing, the sounds around you, and all physical sensations.
  - Observe what you feel, see, and hear without judging it.
  - Continue to focus on each breath, in and out.
  - When intrusive thoughts enter your mind, let them go without judging them or yourself.
  - Return your focus to your breathing.
- *Humor.* Watch a funny movie or television program or read an amusing book.
- *Self-soothing strategies.* These involve the five senses:
  - Sight (look at something pleasant).
  - Taste (prepare and eat good food).

- Smell (buy fragrant flowers or use a favorite scented lotion).
- Touch (wear soft, comfortable clothing or get a massage).
- Hearing (listen to calming music or nature).

- *Routine.* Try to maintain a regular schedule and stay organized. This is a useful strategy for many people who have mood disorders. Begin in one or more of the following ways:
  - Prioritize what you have to do. Do this by keeping lists and an agenda (paper or electronic).
  - Break large tasks down into small steps.
  - Include pleasurable activities and positive events in your day.
  - Keep up with your friends and family.
- *Manage life's little daily stressors.* Prioritize your day, keep a to-do list, and write things down.

Occasionally, irritability becomes such a strong force that it leads the person who has depression to feel out of control. She may seem argumentative and turn to excesses of work, reckless driving, spending, alcohol or substance abuse, or sexual activity. This pattern is more frequently seen in men and adolescents. If this applies to your family member, it requires your utmost patience. It's a time for you to maintain stability, a steady routine, and structure at home. You may need to set expectations and limits on her behavior and remove any alcohol from the home. You may face resistance. Try to remain calm and firm and don't cave in.

DIMINISHED INTEREST OR PLEASURE

Depression may have led your family member to lose interest in her life or things that previously gave her pleasure. They may now seem bland and a waste of time and effort. Work, school, friends, hobbies, sports—why bother? She may prefer to spend time alone, on the sofa watching television, or in her room staring at the wall. Try to engage her in those activities she once enjoyed in small steps and at a pace she can handle now. She doesn't have to actually enjoy the experience; just trying it is enough for now. For example, if she used to like bicycling, you might say, "The weather's great today, and I'd really like to get outside. I'd love it if you would join me for a short ride. We could aim for the old ice cream stand." She may or may not respond positively to this approach on any given day.

Try not to set the bar too high, but don't give up either. The underlying theory is that *action precedes motivation.* This means that your family member or friend should not wait to feel interested or motivated before taking action or joining in an activity. Once she begins to do something, the drive to do it will eventually follow and gain momentum.

You might ask her to identify or list things she is interested in or used to enjoy. Then try to provide opportunities for her to participate in them. If you provide the opportunity, she may be more likely to engage in the activity. If she likes the family dog, you might ask her to do you a favor and take the dog for a walk. This may help her experience the pleasure of being outside, being with the dog, and helping you. See table 3.5 on page 63, Pleasurable Activities, for examples that your loved one might think of doing. Eventually, she may do some of these on her own.

Action precedes motivation.

How to deal with *anhedonia*, the lack of interest in life that comes with depression, is illustrated in this story about Ana. Here, a little perseverance, and taking very small steps, can help to turn things around. Eventually, your loved one will find the strength and motivation to return to some, if not all, of her daily routines, self-care habits, and previously enjoyed activities.

Ana is an 18-year-old high school senior who first experienced symptoms of depression about eight months ago. She was sad all the time, more irritable than usual, and not interested in food or in doing the after-school activities that she always enjoyed. Ana's school grades started to slip, which bothered her, but she had no energy and could not focus and concentrate on her studies. All she wanted to do was sleep 18 hours a day, and her parents and friends could not get her out of her room. Ana felt worthless, a loser, and saw no hope for improvement.

Ana's parents dragged her to first see their family doctor, then to a talk therapist to try to get her back to her usual self. The therapist offered her one piece of advice, a short phrase that resonated with Ana: action precedes motivation. *This meant that she would keep trying to do things even when she didn't feel like it. Ana wasn't sure if she had enough physical or emotional energy to do this, and she didn't quite know if that would restore her motivation and interest in previous activities, but she thought she would try with the help of her family and therapist. She trusted her therapist, who said that her interest, desire, and motivation to do things would gradually return once she got started. But getting started was the difficult part!*

So, each morning when Ana awoke facing a dark and gloomy day of depression, she made herself think of one thing that she would just try to do anyway despite how lousy or tired she felt. The first few days it was to take a shower and put on some clean clothes. Ana was surprised to find that she could actually do those things, and that she felt better afterward. Next, she advanced to joining the family for dinner instead of not eating or staying in her room in bed. Ana found that to be a challenge, requiring more energy than she imagined, for she had to show up and present herself to others, and try to pay attention to the small talk. But she tried it again and again, on most nights, even though she didn't really want to, and eventually she sensed that she preferred family dinner to solitude.

Then Ana's best friend, Claudia, came to visit and encouraged her to get outside to take a walk around the block. "No way," thought Ana. "This is too much!" But she did it anyway, and soon she was out walking the family dog by herself and kicking a soccer ball in the backyard with Claudia. The more she did, the easier it became and the more she was able to do and eventually wanted to do. Motivation was beginning to return, and that was encouraging.

CHANGES IN APPETITE OR WEIGHT

If your family member or friend has depression, her appetite may change. She may want to eat all the time, hungry or not, or she may have no interest in food. This could cause her to eat either too much or too little, leading to an unintentional weight gain or loss of five or more pounds over two or more weeks. This adds to depression and a negative body image. She may be eating fast food or junk food. Poor eating habits can also have an impact on the functioning of her body and brain and her level of fatigue. Try to promote healthy, balanced meals for your family member and encourage her to follow a healthy eating plan without skipping meals or relying on fast food. Keep unhealthy snacks out of the house and set a good example when at home or eating out. Do it together: make a grocery list, take her food shopping with you so that she can choose healthy foods that appeal to her, and enlist her help in preparing the meals.

For help with healthy meal preparation, the US Department of Agriculture (USDA) provides an online list of Dietary Guidelines for Americans at www.dietaryguidelines.gov. See table 3.2 on page 52 for more information.

DIFFICULTY SLEEPING

Problems with sleep are common in many people who have unipolar or bipolar depression. She may experience difficulty falling asleep or staying asleep, she may have fragmented sleep, or she may wake up too early in the morning. She may sleep much longer than usual, with additional naps in the middle of the day, or sleep very little. All of these patterns can be symptoms of depression, and she should speak with her doctor about them. If she is experiencing the mania or hypomania of bipolar disorder, she might feel energized and sense no need for sleep or have fragmented sleep. Healthy sleep habits, called Sleep Hygiene guidelines, from the American Academy of Sleep Medicine are listed in table 3.1 on page 51 (www.sleepeducation.com /essentials-in-sleep/healthy-sleep-habits). This set of guidelines is helpful, and it's important for all of us to follow the guidelines, particularly someone who has a mood disorder.

PHYSICAL RESTLESSNESS OR SLOWING DOWN

Some people who have depression may experience an unusual form of restlessness and agitation, with a constant inner urge to move about and not sit still. This differs from anxiety. Others find they are physically slowed down, which is not the same as fatigue. Some describe it as feeling like an elephant is sitting on them or they are moving through molasses. If your family member or friend finds either of these to be true, she should discuss this with her doctor. A regular physical exercise routine may help.

FATIGUE

During an episode of depression, your loved one may feel tired and worn out. Such fatigue can be physical, mental, and emotional. Physical fatigue can include a loss of energy, tiredness, and a reduced ability to exercise. Mental fatigue can involve dulled thinking, problems with focus and attention, or difficulty concentrating. Emotional fatigue frequently involves a lack of motivation, apathy, or weariness. Fatigue can be a symptom of depression, a side effect of medications, or related to insomnia or poor sleep patterns. Make sure your family member or friend discusses the fatigue with her doctor.

If fatigue is a factor in your family member, try to encourage her to stick to the Basics of Mental Health. This means keeping regular sleep hours, with a goal of seven to eight hours of sleep per night but not more. Many people who have depression find it helpful to follow a healthy and balanced diet, with adequate fluid intake (eight glasses of nonalcoholic fluid per day).

Regular physical exercise helps as well. You might become your family member's or friend's exercise partner by going out with her for a moderate to brisk walk around the block several times a week. This may seem contrary to what you or she may think: How in the world can such a tired person go out and exercise? However, regular exercise is often quite helpful in reversing the symptoms of fatigue. She may be pleasantly surprised at its positive effect.

FEELINGS OF WORTHLESSNESS OR GUILT

You may find that your family member or friend with depression experiences feelings of worthlessness or guilt without cause. Your best response to her assertions of worthlessness is to provide active listening and empathic responses. You might begin with asking, "Why do you think you're feeling [worthless, guilty]?" Try to get her to share the reasons that are driving her thoughts. You may find that distorted negative thoughts are behind her feelings of worthlessness (see chapter 8). If so, explore with her what is fact and what is distorted thinking. You might ask, "I hear you feel you're worthless in life. That must be very painful. Can you tell me more about what makes you feel this way?" Then help her try to focus on the facts. Remind her of her past successes.

If your friend or family member feels worthless at work, you might say, "I remember last month when you received praise for your part in getting the project done ahead of schedule. How has their opinion of you changed since then?" Your goal is to bring up prior successes that counteract her feelings. The Evidence For and Against exercise (see table 8.1 on page 119) in chapter 8 may also be useful.

If your family member or friend feels guilty about something she had little control over, you might ask about the reasons for her feelings and the facts behind them: "What about this situation is making you feel guilty? Do you think you did something to contribute to the outcome?" Find out her level of participation in the event and whether she is carrying the burden for someone else. With no strong facts to back up her feelings of guilt, she is more likely to drop that emotion.

DIMINISHED ABILITY TO THINK, FOCUS, OR CONCENTRATE

Trouble concentrating is one of the most common symptoms of depression. It can be particularly frustrating for your family member or friend if she uses her mind every day to perform complex tasks or to make major decisions. Focus problems may include difficulty reading and with conversations or recreational activities such as watching a movie or television. It can be annoying and may interfere with her ability to function at her best on a daily basis. Try to help your family member find acceptable work-arounds to compensate. Here are some of the ways you might suggest that help her meet these challenges:

- Write things down on sticky notes or in a paper or an electronic notebook carried daily.
- Use an agenda (paper or electronic) to keep track of meetings and appointments.
- Take notes during group and individual meetings and appointments. Ask permission first.
- Break large tasks into small steps and complete them one by one.
- Focus on one thing at a time. Avoid multitasking.
- Read slowly and reread a paragraph as necessary. Take notes if needed.
- Watch a short television show rather than a full-length movie for entertainment.
- Learn to say no. A person who has depression may need to accept some limitations in what she can realistically do right now. She should be careful in what and how much she takes on. This includes learning to say no to requests for her time when she feels overwhelmed. It may also mean working or going to school on a part-time basis or taking a temporary leave of absence.

THOUGHTS OF DEATH OR SUICIDE, OR A SUICIDE PLAN

Some of those who experience depression, including perhaps your family member or friend, may have thoughts of death or suicide. These may be specific, such as wanting to kill himself, or they may come out as a vague statement of not wanting to "be around." He may talk about not wanting to be a burden to others, having no reason to live, or feeling unbearable emotional pain. You may notice a drastic change in his behavior or how he takes care of himself. Your loved one may show a loss of interest, withdrawal and isolation from others, changes in sleep or diet, or substance or alcohol use. He may appear depressed, irritable, or anxious. He may have recently experienced a major loss in his life. The Warning Signs of Suicide are presented in table 10.1; Risk Factors for Suicide are presented in table 10.2 on page 142. Suicidal thoughts may come and go. If you hear any comments like those described, take them very seriously.

> Suicidal thoughts are a psychiatric emergency.

If your family member or friend shows any sign of a plan or intent to commit suicide, call for professional help immediately by dialing 9-1-1, his mental health provider, or bring him to the closest Emergency Department for evaluation. In the meantime, remove anything he might use for this purpose (pills or weapons, for example), and do not leave him alone. See chapter 10 for more on this.

10

When Someone Is Suicidal

SUICIDE

The most severe form of depression can lead someone to consider self-harm or suicide. This may or may not apply to your family member or friend at some point, but it's worth knowing about. Suicide is usually considered an impulsive act in a troubled person who sees no way to change his or her painful circumstances. Suicidal thoughts and acts happen when his deep emotional pain or a stressor exceeds his ability to cope with that pain. In the chaos and anguish of the moment, it is often not possible for a person to reach the logical part of his brain to change these troubling and distorted thoughts. A suicidal act often surprises family members and close friends because the person is not perceived as impulsive and hides their emotional pain deep inside.

Mental health clinicians have observed differences in the thought patterns of those who no longer want to continue living, which they classify as active suicidal ideation, passive suicidal ideation, chronic and acute. These are defined as follows. A person who no longer wishes to live and has made specific plans for his death has *active suicidal ideation*. A person who no longer wants to be around anymore but has not made any plans has *passive suicidal ideation*. This is still considered serious and can rapidly become "active" if and when major life stressors occur in a person unable to think clearly and logically because of illness or substance abuse. *Chronic* means that it has been going on for a long time, usually several months. *Acute* refers to recent onset. You as a support person and family member are not expected to detect these differences in your loved one; even though you may have heard his suicidal thoughts before, I recommend that you act on each time as an urgent call for help and take steps to have him evaluated.

> Suicide is a tragic consequence of the thought disturbances in a mood disorder.

Suicide is one of the greatest tragedies in the United States and in the world. In 2018, it was reported that 48,341 persons committed suicide in the United States (American Foundation for Suicide Prevention [AFSP] 2020; data from the Centers for Disease Control and Prevention [CDC]). Of those, just over three-quarters were male (77.9% male, 22.1% female). The highest numbers were in middle-age white males and men over age 85. It is the second leading cause of death in those aged 15 to 34 (CDC 2016), peaking in adolescents, adults, and the elderly.

Suicide rates have been rising in the Unites States, increasing by approximately 25 to 30 percent from 1999 to 2016 in all states but one. Firearms were the most common method used (50.6%), followed by suffocation (27.7%) and poisoning (13.9%). In 2018, there were 1.4 million suicide attempts (AFSP, 2020) in the United States. In keeping with the numbers showing women's higher depression rates, females made 1.4 times more suicide attempts than males; however, males died by suicide 3.5 times more often.

In the United States, military veterans die from suicide about one-and-a-half times more often than those who have not served, resulting in approximately 20 suicide deaths per day among veterans. Reviews of mental health care and suicide prevention programs at VA centers found that veterans often receive good care there; however, about 70 percent of veterans do not use the VA system. Why is this? High rates of homelessness, traumatic brain injury, post-traumatic stress, and military culture that resists mental health care treatment and emphasizes perseverance and an "I can do it" mentality are all contributing factors. Firearms are used in the majority of veteran suicides, as gun ownership is high for that group.

> Suicide rates have been rising in the Unites States.

Globally, the exact rates of suicide are difficult to obtain. An estimated 800,000 persons worldwide die from suicide each year (World Health Organization 2018). Suicide varies within and between countries. This is partly due to economic conditions and cultural differences, disruption of traditional cultural and family supports, areas of lower socioeconomic status, and increased alcohol and substance use.

The numbers for those who have tried to seriously harm themselves or attempt suicide without completion are also hard to get so they may not be accurate. While many suicide attempts go unreported or untreated, surveys suggest that at least one million people harm themselves each year in the United States. The CDC gathers information from hospitals on nonfatal injuries that occur from self-harm. In 2015, there were 575,000 visits to a hospital in the United States for injuries due to self-harm (AFSP 2019). According to the 2017 Youth Risk Behavior Survey (from the CDC), approximately 7.4 percent of teens in grades 9–12 made one suicide attempt in the preceding 12 months, and girls were twice as likely as boys to act. The percentage of youth who reported persistent feelings of sadness or hopelessness increased from 29 percent in 2007 to 32 percent in 2017.

The average cost of suicide is $1.3 million per life lost, 97 percent due to lost productivity (Suicide Prevention Resource Center 2019). The cost of suicide to society in the United States is estimated at $70 billion per year for combined suicide and self-injury, including medical and work-loss costs (CDC 2018).

More than half of those who died by suicide did not have a known, diagnosed mental health condition at the time of their death (CDC 2018). In contrast, the AFSP discovered some flaws in the CDC data collection process; they report that, when examined in more depth, 90 percent of those who commit suicide had a diagnosable mental health condition at the time of their death (AFSP 2020).

Suicide is not due to any one thing. The CDC 2018 report notes that many factors contribute to taking one's life: (1) relationship problems or loss, (2) substance use issues, (3) physical health problems, (4) job or financial/money stress, (5) other life stressors, (6) recent or impending life crises, (7) legal problems, and (8) housing stress.

Anyone struggling with serious lifestyle problems is at risk. Cultural attitudes may also play a part. Those without a known mental health condition, according to the report, were more likely to be male and belong to a racial or ethnic minority and less likely to seek help. While school bullying has

Suicide is rarely caused by a single factor.

been a recent major concern in adolescents, it has not been proven to be a *direct* cause of suicide (CDC 2014) although current thinking suggests there is a relationship and that it has a significant impact on suicidal thoughts and behaviors (Lardier 2016). One theory that attempts to explain why a person would perform a suicidal act suggests that suicidal behavior involves a vulnerability or predisposition in the person (from a previous trauma or adversity, family genetics, hopelessness, substance use, recent major loss) who then experiences a major stress (acute psychiatric illness, interpersonal problem, life event, etc.) that triggers the impulsive suicidal act.

Many experts have offered other theories of suicide in an attempt to understand it, yet there is no one model that fits all persons and situations. Some of the ideas presented include:

- hopelessness
- perceived burdensomeness
- absence of meaningful connections
- unbearable psychological pain
- rigid thinking
- inability to cope with problems and losses

- damaged interpersonal relationship
- loss or abandonment
- rejection
- damaged self-image
- falling short of standards or expectations
- setbacks
- self-blame
- reckless behaviors and irrational thought

Some age groups may be more vulnerable to contemplating self-harm or suicide. Many adolescents and teenagers have a difficult time during this phase of their lives. They feel pressure to succeed in school and to fit in with their peers. Some struggle with self-esteem and self-doubt. This age group also exhibits a fair amount of impulsive behavior. In the older adult age group, persons may face loneliness, loss of friends and family, physical impairments that limit their lifestyle, medical problems and chronic pain, retirement, or loss of independence and purpose.

Suicidal thoughts and behaviors of any kind are considered a psychiatric emergency. They require immediate response. If your family member shows any signs of suicide intent, consider it an emergency and follow the steps outlined next to have your loved one evaluated.

WARNING SIGNS OF SUICIDE

Keep an eye out for the Warning Signs of Suicide in your loved one who has depression (AFSP 2019; table 10.1). These are distinct changes in what your family member or friend says, does, or thinks that are noticed by you or others. They are signs for major concern. Warning Signs of Suicide include talking about death or suicide, having a suicide plan, feeling severe hopelessness, experiencing a drastic change in behavior, withdrawing from her normal activities, losing interest in people or social activities, and more.

She might mutter, "I wish I hadn't been born," "I'd be better off dead," or "Everybody would be better off without me." She might start giving away her prized possessions, withdraw from friends and family, or use or increase her intake of alcohol or street drugs. Pay close attention to these statements and actions; consider them an alert that she's serious about harming herself.

The following story about Lee gives us a sense of how a major stress and loss in life, combined with a feeling of rejection and isolation, without social support, can lead to depression and suicidal thoughts in a vulnerable person who is unable to access her previously helpful coping skills.

TABLE 10.1. **Warning Signs of Suicide**
Changes in talking Talks about killing self or having a suicide plan Believes he or she has no reason to live Concerned about being a burden to others Has unbearable emotional pain *Changes in behavior* Increased use of alcohol or drugs Looks for a way to kill self Acts recklessly Withdraws from activities and life Isolates self from family and friends Sleeps too much or too little Says goodbye to others Gives away possessions Behaves aggressively *Changes in mood* Depression Loss of interest Anger, rage, irritability Humiliation Anxiety

Source: According to the American Foundation for Suicide Prevention (AFSP, www.afsp.org) www.afsp.org/preventing-suicide-warning-signs, accessed March 2019.

Lee is a 50-year-old woman recently divorced from her husband of 23 years who up and ran off with a much younger woman. This was quite devastating. Lee's family had been her life, but now their two sons are grown and live in different states—one still in college, one working—and she lives alone. Since her divorce, her social situation has greatly changed: she had to stop her previous social activities, many of "their" friends stopped calling anymore and she feels quite isolated, without social support. She has fewer financial resources and is having financial difficulties. Lee was forced to move from her quiet home and neighborhood, where she knew most people, to a noisy apartment quite a distance away where nobody even says hello. Her ex-husband is refusing to support her with alimony. Lee's attempts at finding a job have been unsuccessful so far, since she had been out of the work force for two decades raising her family and has no current skills.

Lee has been feeling sad, tearful, unloved, and recently has been feel-ing hopeless and depressed with trouble sleeping and eating. She's been having a lot of right knee pain lately from an old injury and has stopped her usual fitness walks. She worries constantly about her future—how she can afford to live and what her days will be like. Right now it does not feel as though her two sons are connected to her. They seem to prefer their father, and she is heartbroken. At night, she has taken to drinking up to a bottle of wine by herself, feeling lonely and rejected. Her previous coping skills, useful during difficult times, don't seem to be available to her, and she doesn't really care.

Last night Lee was in great emotional pain and started to wonder if anybody would even miss her if she were gone, believing that they would all be better off without her around. She did not want to be a burden to her children and could not see a future ahead of her. She reached for a handful of pills that she had been saving up, which to her seemed as though they would bring permanent relief, and just then an old friend rang her doorbell and was able to problem-solve with her and get her to immediate profes-sional, lifesaving mental health care.

RISK FACTORS FOR SUICIDE

There are some Risk Factors for Suicide that you should be aware of (iden-tified by CDC; National Suicide Prevention Lifeline). These are factors in a person's life that *could* increase the chance he might consider or attempt suicide. The risk factors for suicide only point out that a person has a higher likelihood for suicide based on his life history. They are not a guarantee that suicide will happen. Risk factors are not the same as the Warning Signs of Suicide, which are distinct changes in a person's behavior or speech.

Some of the identified risk factors are listed in table 10.2. These include a previous suicide attempt; a family history of suicide; a history of trauma, abuse, or early life adversity; a history of alcohol and substance abuse; hope-lessness; male gender; living alone or in social isolation; and many others. There is some suggestion that veterans, particularly those suffering with post-traumatic stress disorder, or PTSD, may be at increased risk. There is conflicted data about whether cyberbullying in adolescents and teenagers puts them at increased risk; the current thinking is that it may. Any of these risk factors may or may not apply to your family member or friend.

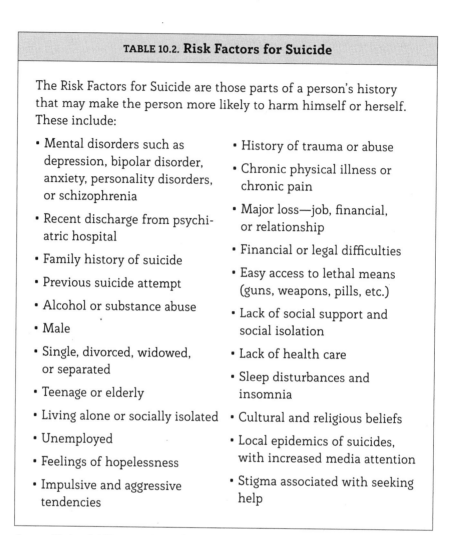

TABLE 10.2. Risk Factors for Suicide

The Risk Factors for Suicide are those parts of a person's history that may make the person more likely to harm himself or herself. These include:

- Mental disorders such as depression, bipolar disorder, anxiety, personality disorders, or schizophrenia
- Recent discharge from psychiatric hospital
- Family history of suicide
- Previous suicide attempt
- Alcohol or substance abuse
- Male
- Single, divorced, widowed, or separated
- Teenage or elderly
- Living alone or socially isolated
- Unemployed
- Feelings of hopelessness
- Impulsive and aggressive tendencies
- History of trauma or abuse
- Chronic physical illness or chronic pain
- Major loss—job, financial, or relationship
- Financial or legal difficulties
- Easy access to lethal means (guns, weapons, pills, etc.)
- Lack of social support and social isolation
- Lack of health care
- Sleep disturbances and insomnia
- Cultural and religious beliefs
- Local epidemics of suicides, with increased media attention
- Stigma associated with seeking help

Sources: National Alliance on Mental Illness (NAMI), www.nami.org; Centers for Disease Control and Prevention (CDC), www.cdc.gov/violenceprevention/suicide; National Suicide Prevention Lifeline, www.suicidepreventionlifeline.org/learn/riskfactors.

WHAT TO DO

Your first response when your family member or friend mentions harming himself is to sit down with him and discuss his feelings and thoughts on death and suicide. Stay neutral and calm. Be supportive and empathetic. Listen with your full attention and encourage him to speak openly about these painful things. Be aware that the person may have beliefs and attitudes about suicide that differ from your own (for example, your beliefs that suicide is wrong or his beliefs that it's a rational option) and try to separate out your own thoughts and remain neutral.

It can be scary to hear about suicide and to talk about it. If you are unable to have this conversation, call for professional help immediately. If you feel you can speak about it, take a deep breath and stay calm during this conversation. You can be most helpful if you sit and listen to your family member's or friend's thoughts of self-harm and any suicidal thoughts or plans he may have.

Don't underestimate your abilities to help a person who is suicidal. One way to start is to say, "I've been very concerned about you lately. Have you ever thought about harming yourself or wishing that you weren't here?" Let her know you care and that she's not alone. Do your best to listen.

If she mentions thoughts of suicide, it's *not* helpful to respond quickly with "No, you don't! How could you possibly think that way?" Try to use supportive words that are not perceived as judgmental or dismissive. Don't say, "You're not thinking of doing anything stupid, are you?" Don't use guilt or threats to pressure her out of it ("It's a sin." "You'll go to hell." "You'll ruin our lives."). Never dare her to do it, interrupt with your own stories, or minimize her painful problems.

> Suicide is a psychiatric emergency.

Instead, ask her directly and gently if she has specific details or a suicide plan: "Do you have a plan?" "What is it?" "When?" and "Do you have what you need to carry out your plan?" Find out if she is hearing voices and if the voices are directing her to take action. Know that the lack of a plan does not guarantee her safety. Mental Health First Aid has created a helpful guideline for assessing suicidal thoughts and behaviors, and I have included a link to their page in the list of resources.

If your family member shows any indication of suicide intent or a plan, take it seriously. Call for professional help immediately by dialing 9-1-1 or her mental health provider. The goal is to keep your loved one safe and have her evaluated by an experienced mental health professional. In the meantime, remove anything (pills, knives, firearms) she might use for this purpose from her environment. Do not leave her alone.

It is often reassuring for your family member to hear that while thoughts of suicide may seem real and urgent, she should not believe them or act on them. Encourage her to recognize that it's the depression driving her thoughts. Suicidal thoughts are wayward thoughts, not facts, and will last only a short time. Our emotions are constantly shifting; they are not permanent or fixed, even if she seems to return to the same familiar ones repeatedly. Although emotions are driven by strong urges, they *will* change and will pass in time.

Some people fear that speaking of suicide with a person who has depression may make the situation worse. But having this conversation will *not* encourage her to take action. Asking about suicide and encouraging your family member or friend to get help does not increase the risk of suicide. Rather, it signals to her that you care and gives her an opportunity to talk about her problems. Talking about it may lower the chance of suicide.

Remind your loved one that the challenge is to get through this time safely, until her (temporarily disorganized) mind is able to manage her problems. Once the urgency has passed, she will have time to work on the problems that brought her to this point. Encourage him to get professional mental health treatment as soon as possible. Don't assume that he will get better on his own. You can help by finding out about available resources for people at risk in his area (see chapter 4).

Know that while you can offer support and provide for safety, you are *not* responsible for the actions of someone else and cannot control what he or she might decide to do. It is impossible for even the best-trained mental health professional to accurately predict what actions every person might take, and often these plans are cleverly hidden from others like you.

Also know that the suicidal person may become angry with you and feel betrayed because you interrupted his self-harm plans. Try not to take this personally, including any hurtful words that may come your way. In the long run, speaking up and taking action against suicide is in his best interest. It is better to have him angry with you than to lose him permanently.

SUICIDE PREVENTION

Once you know the life factors that put your family member or friend at risk, you can take the following steps to prevent his or her suicide. First, ensure she receives effective evaluation and medical care for her mental, physical, or substance use disorders with a combination of medical and mental health treatments. You may want to help her arrange these treatments since the telephone calls and paperwork to schedule appointments can be an effort. She may also need a referral for these treatments from her primary care physician, depending on her type of health insurance plan.

Second, make sure she has no access to lethal means of suicide: pills, firearms, knives, and other weapons in the home. This means going through the house from top to bottom and removing anything she might be able to use or that might tempt her or put her at risk.

Third, and most important, provide her with support and a strong connection to you, her friends and family, and her community. This includes support through her ongoing medical and mental health providers. A sense of social connectedness can make a big difference. Encourage her to learn and use skills in problem solving, resolving conflicts, and handling her problems in a nonviolent way (see chapter 9). In addition, for many people, spiritual and religious beliefs that validate the need for self-preservation and discourage self-harm have been very useful.

EMERGENCY RESPONSE

Suicide is a psychiatric emergency. If you suspect your family member or friend is suicidal, this is the time to be firm and pick up the phone to one of the following resources for his safety and evaluation:

- His therapist, psychiatrist, family doctor or primary care physician, or school counselor
- In the USA: call the National Suicide Prevention Lifeline at 800-273-8255
- In the United States: call the Samaritans at 877-870-4673
- In the United States: call the Veterans' Crisis Line: 800-273-8255
- In the United Kingdom and Ireland: call the Samaritans at 116 123 or +44(0)08457909090
- In Australia: call Lifeline Australia at 13 11 14
- In Argentina: call +5402234930430
- In Austria: call 017133374
- In Brazil: call CVV National Association at (081)3231–4141 plus multiple numbers online
- In Canada: call 5147234000 (Montreal) plus multiple numbers online
- In China: call 08008101117 or (21)63798990
- In France: call 0145394000
- In Germany: call 08001810771
- In Israel: call 11201 or 97298891333
- In Italy: call 800860022 or 199284284
- In Japan: call 81(0)352869090 or 81(0)643954343
- In Mexico: call 5255102550
- In New Zealand: call (64)033531136 plus multiple numbers online
- In Spain: call 914590050
- In South Africa: call 0861322322 plus multiple numbers online
- In other countries: call your local helpline listed on www.suicide.org

In addition to reaching out to your loved one, follow these critical steps:

- Have him promise not to do anything right now.
- See that he avoids illicit drugs and alcohol.
- Follow his safety plan, such as the Action Plan for Relapse Prevention.
- Remind him of those in his life who love him and would feel grief and anguish in his absence—do it in a way without laying on guilt!
- Don't allow him to isolate; don't leave him alone.

If you think it can't wait, call 9-1-1 or take him to your local hospital Emergency Department for evaluation. The mental health response team will then decide if and how best to act. Sometimes having suicidal thoughts or desires means he has to be admitted to the hospital until the crisis passes. That's okay. He will be safe there and evaluated by mental health professionals who will modify his treatment plan as needed.

Mood Disorders and Addictions

DUAL DIAGNOSIS

You may find that your loved one has become involved in using alcohol, illegal drugs, or other substances to buffer his or her deep emotional pain. Substance use may occur on an occasional basis or become a regular problem he cannot control. Some people who experience a mental health condition may turn to alcohol or other drugs to self-medicate; their way of relieving their mental health symptoms. However, this is not an effective strategy and research shows that alcohol and other drugs worsen the symptoms of mental illness.

Dual diagnosis is a term that describes those who experience a mental illness and a substance use disorder at the same time. Either of these two conditions can also occur first—substance use or mental illness—when they are referred to as *co-occurring* disorders.

According to a 2014 National Survey on Drug Use and Health, 7.9 million people in the United States experience both a mental disorder and a substance use disorder at the same time. More than half of those people—4.1 million—are men.

You might wonder why these two disorders can be linked? Predisposing genetic factors may make a person susceptible to having both addiction and a mental health disorder. In addition, environmental factors in your loved one's life—stress, trauma (physical or emotional), and early exposure to drugs—are often overlapping and can influence the development of addiction and other mental illnesses. And, yes, drug addiction is a mental illness that changes the brain in specific ways.

> Dual diagnosis refers to those who have a mental illness and substance use disorder simultaneously.

The substance most commonly used in excess or abused is alcohol, followed by marijuana (cannabis) and cocaine. Males aged 18 to 44 are at greatest risk. Mental illness and substance abuse are biologically—and physiologically—based and have both mental and physical effects; they are true medical conditions and the person needs professional help to deal with them. Substance use complicates almost every aspect of care for the person who has a mental illness. It is especially complex and difficult to manage.

Cannabis (marijuana) is the most commonly abused used drug in the world, and it has a number of side effects. Among US adolescents, 20.9 percent report use in the past month, and 7 percent of US high school seniors report daily or near-daily cannabis use. The numbers are fairly similar globally. There is known to be an increased and earlier onset of psychosis with cannabis use. *Psychosis* is an altered condition of the mind where the person loses his sense of reality and may have hallucinations, delusions (fixed false beliefs), and disordered thoughts and speech. Psychosis can be caused by some medications, alcohol or drug abuse, or a mental illness, including some forms of depression and schizophrenia.

> Alcohol, marijuana, and cocaine are the most commonly abused substances in the world.

A combined review of many scientific studies (a systematic review and meta-analysis) confirmed that, when cannabis is used in adolescence, the risk of developing depression and suicidal thoughts and behavior in later life increases (Gobbi 2019). Girls seem more likely to develop depression in later life following teenage cannabis use. Side effects include decreased achievement in school, dropping out of school and studies, the potential for addiction, adverse birth outcomes in the offspring of mothers with cannabis habits, and neuropsychological decline. Some of this is because the adolescent brain is still developing, and psychotropic drugs may alter the physiologic and neurologic development of the brain.

A report in *Lancet Psychiatry* showed daily cannabis use is strongly linked to the risk of developing psychosis (DiForti et al. 2019). Psychosis is an altered state of mind with a loss of reality. The risk of psychosis is greater when a stronger or more potent form of marijuana is used (high potency is defined as greater than 10% THC concentration). This study looked at data from 901 persons aged 10 to 64 who had first-time psychosis across 11 sites in Europe and Brazil. The findings varied by region, and were most pronounced in Amsterdam and London, where high potency cannabis is widely available as compared to Italy, France or Spain. For example, in Amsterdam, daily cannabis use was associated with 43.8 percent of first-time psychosis cases and 50.3 percent of psychosis cases for high potency use.

Substance *addiction* is a more severe problem than substance *use or abuse*. Addiction involves regular use in higher amounts than substance use or abuse. In addiction, the person is often unable to stop once using starts, despite the negative consequences or poor health it may cause. Addiction implies physiologic dependence, tolerance, and withdrawal symptoms after stopping drug use.

SYMPTOMS

Someone who has a problem with addiction or dual diagnosis may change her behavior in many ways from her usual self. In addition to the physical influence of the drug, symptoms of substance use or abuse disorder may include:

- Withdrawal from friends and family
- Sudden changes in behavior
- Using substances under dangerous social conditions or settings
- Engaging in risky behaviors
- Loss of control over use of substances
- Developing a high tolerance for the same dose of the drug
- Withdrawal symptoms
- Feeling like you need a drug to be able to function

What Should You Look For in Your Loved One?

Many people who have a substance use or abuse problem try to hide it from their friends and families in clever ways. Be on the lookout for changes in behavior:

- Sudden financial problems
- Failure to meet obligations, such as school or work
- Reckless activities (driving while intoxicated)
- Legal troubles (getting arrested)
- Valuables disappearing from the household
- Spending a long time in the bathroom
- Dilated or pinpoint pupils
- Needle marks on the skin
- Drug paraphernalia found in the house (needles, syringes, tourniquets, etc.)

Ed is a 45-year-old financially successful businessman who has a history of major depression and substance abuse. He began with using marijuana in college, along with social alcohol on the weekends and then advanced to cocaine use and alcohol binge drinking. Major depression became apparent about five years ago. He did not seek professional psychiatric treatment until he was forced to by the courts after a DUI arrest. However, he did not stick with treatment for long.

Ed's marriage is on the rocks, and his business partners have lost their patience with his behavior. They note he often comes in late to work, is not pulling his weight, and is failing to meet his obligations with clients. He seems to be withdrawn and isolated. His wife, Meredith, sees changes in his mood with periods of extreme irritability and agitation, insomnia, risk taking, and feeling worthless and hopeless. She fears for their financial security and wants to file for a legal separation and keep him away from their two teenage children until he can get clean and sober, with his depression treated. But she is skeptical because he has been in rehab twice before without long-term success. This has had a major impact on Meredith, the children, and the family. Ed does not see that he has a real problem because he considers drinking and snorting with clients is part of customer service! He is willing to enter treatment, though, because he does not want to lose his family or his affluent lifestyle.

Meredith has planned an intervention in which she, his brother and sister-in-law, and two of Ed's (sober) friends will sit down with him and describe what he is like now, what they see he is doing to himself, and how he is different from his healthy self. They will remind Ed of their love and concern for him and offer him their full support; however, and this time, they will intervene using a tough love approach. Meredith will present her plan for legal separation as a realistic option if he is not able to participate successfully in an integrated treatment plan that includes detox, inpatient rehabilitation, intensive psychotherapy, and medication therapy as needed.

TREATMENT

The most effective treatment for dual diagnosis is an *integrated intervention,* when a person receives care for both diagnosed mental illness and substance abuse at the same time. With this treatment, people support each other as they learn about the role alcohol and illegal substances have in their lives. They learn social skills, how to replace substance use with new thoughts and behaviors, and receive concrete help for situations related to their mental illness.

Treatment for dual diagnosis is complex and not easy to do. It is also more expensive. Persons with both mental health and substance abuse conditions have treatment costs that are 61 percent higher, and total medical care costs that are 44 percent higher than for those who have depression alone.

Stages of Treatment

Your loved one will have to undergo several stages of the treatment process. These are not easy. Your role is to be supportive, help him to complete each stage and to return to treatment as needed if slipups occur.

Detoxification. This is the first stage in which the person stops taking the substance he is abusing and may experience uncomfortable symptoms of withdrawal. Inpatient detoxification is generally more effective than outpatient to achieve initial sobriety and safety. During inpatient detoxification, trained medical staff monitor a person 24/7 for up to seven days. The staff may administer tapering amounts of the substance or its medical alternative to wean a person off and lessen the effects of withdrawal.

Inpatient rehabilitation. A person experiencing a mental illness and dangerous, dependent patterns of substance use may benefit from an inpatient rehabilitation center where he can receive medical and mental health care 24/7. These treatment centers provide therapy, support, medication, and health services to treat the substance use disorder and its underlying causes.

Supportive housing. These are residential treatment centers like group homes or sober houses that may help people who are newly sober or trying to avoid relapse. These centers provide some support and independence. Sober homes have sometimes been criticized for offering varying levels of quality care because licensed professionals do not typically run them. You need to do some research when selecting a treatment setting.

Psychotherapy. Psychotherapy is a large part of an effective dual diagnosis treatment plan. Cognitive behavioral therapy helps people with dual diagnosis learn how to cope and change ineffective patterns of thinking and behavior, which may influence the risk of substance use.

Medications. Medications are useful for treating mental illnesses. Certain medications can also help people experiencing substance use disorders ease withdrawal symptoms during the detoxification process and help to promote recovery.

Self-help and support groups. Dealing with a dual diagnosis can feel challenging and isolating. Support groups allow members to share frustrations, celebrate successes, find referrals for specialists, identify community resources, and swap recovery tips. They also provide a space for forming healthy friendships filled with encouragement to stay clean. Here are some groups NAMI recommends:

- Double Trouble in Recovery: a 12-step fellowship for people managing both a mental illness and substance abuse.
- Alcoholics Anonymous and Narcotics Anonymous: 12-step groups for people recovering from alcohol or drug addiction. Neither one alone is sufficient to treat dual diagnosis. One also needs to be receiving expert mental health care. Be sure to find a group that understands the role of mental health treatment in substance recovery.
- Smart Recovery: a non-faith-based sobriety support group for people with a variety of addictions.

For the Parents of a Teen or Young Adult and the Teens with an Affected Parent

You, the parents of a teen or young adult, can often find yourselves in a challenging position when it comes to the emotional health of your child. They are in transition and are trying hard to stand on their own. Most don't want to have a parent hovering, having you know their innermost emotional thoughts, fears, concerns, and presumed failures. Privacy and autonomy (the ability to act on his or her own values and interests without being controlled) are important to them. Yet you want to protect them from the evils and pain of the world and impart your wisdom and hard-earned life lessons to your loved one. It's difficult for parents to give up that role of protector, of keeping their child safe from harm. And every generation has its own unique set of complex problems to navigate—your child's experiences are different from those you had growing up. Despite your best attempts to understand, there is often a chasm in your communication, where your relationship with your teen or young adult may feel broken, and she may just not open up to you or she may appear hostile. Some kids rebel and don't want to live by anyone else's rules; most crave acceptance, fitting in with an urge to be cool.

As Faber and Mazlish (2005) describe so well in their book *How to Talk So Teens Will Listen & Listen So Teens Will Talk*, teenagers need to be able to express their feelings, doubts, fears and explore options in the safety of a family with an adult who will listen nonjudgmentally and help them make responsible decisions. They need help in resisting peer pressure, coping with cliques, cruelties, bullying, fear of rejection, and their longing for acceptance as they travel through the confusion of adolescence. All of this now has to be done in a culture that has become mean, crude, materialistic, highly sexualized and violent, and they feel overwhelmed. This is a difficult time for a young person and his parents.

HOW YOU CAN HELP

You can help by providing a safe home climate using the following tactics. Try to accept and acknowledge his feelings and not dismiss them as unimportant. Avoid the urge some may have, particularly when you're tired, frustrated, and worn out, to ridicule his thoughts or criticize his judgment in haste. Try instead to be open and understanding and accept those thoughts and feelings as valid, even if you disagree at the moment. Listen and let him know he's been heard (see more on this in chapter 7). Acceptance of one's feelings can give comfort and make it easier for your teen to feel understood and cope in life. Teens need a supportive home environment with structure, where they know what to expect from you. Later on you can delicately deal with the distorted content of his thoughts.

> Look for a change in his usual baseline self.

It's difficult for most of us to interpret what's going on in the mind of a teen or young adult. Many of the behaviors commonly associated with adolescence and the transition to young adulthood—moodiness, anger and irritability, social withdrawal—may be signs of depression. But oftentimes normal teen angst or behaviors in growing up can be mistaken for depression. It can be tricky for you to know the difference, to understand whether it's a phase of adolescent behavior or a mental health problem. Most adolescents won't know or won't reach out to ask for help themselves. So, you may feel left out, struggling to figure out how best to help.

Teenagers face extraordinary pressures from peers, school, family, or themselves, while also dealing with changing bodies, including changes in the body's balance of hormones, in a society that emphasizes body image. And they face astonishing pressure to perform and to fit in with others. It's often all played out on social media, with little or no privacy. All of this can contribute to depression. The end result is that a mood disorder in an adolescent, teenage or young adult looks and feels different from that in other age groups.

Try to Keep Things Normal

Treat your adolescent or young adult who has depression as normal as possible. The last thing they want is to be considered odd or treated in a different manner. This involves including her in family activities and holding her to your expectations regarding responsibilities around the house—cleaning her room, doing the dishes or other chores, being cordial to siblings and visitors, going to school and completing homework assignments.

Some teenagers may miss days of school or work or need to take a temporary leave of absence from school until they feel and function better, and that's okay. It's only a pause in the path of her life and is not as devastating as it might initially seem. People often take a gap year or semester for a variety of reasons. As she feels better, she will be able to make up the time. But try to use this judiciously and not allow her to use this as a crutch, missing days of school or homework assignments when it is not seriously needed and she is not in crisis. She will eventually have to make up this school work and there will be added stress and anxiety if these responsibilities pile up in an unmanageable way. It may be helpful to confidentially discuss your teen's current challenges with some of her teachers and create a plan where she can realistically pace herself academically, maintain her self-esteem, and not fall too far behind.

WHAT TO LOOK FOR

Typically, you'll see a change from his usual baseline self. Irritability and agitation is a common feature of depression in an adolescent, sometimes the hallmark symptom. Your teenager might be more withdrawn and isolated, often hiding out in his room. He may now be more secretive about what he does, where he goes and with whom, socializing with kids you've never met perhaps. He may become argumentative and fight with his parents or siblings over minor things.

Daily habits, such as sleeping more, eating different foods or junk foods with a significant weight loss or gain, or not eating, substance use, and social activities, may all change without explanation. There may be a noticeable

- shift in school or work performance,
- change (drop) in grades,
- loss of friends or a new group of friends, or
- change in activities once enjoyed.

Maybe he considers playing soccer to now be too "lame," or he doesn't fit in with the team he once liked and now wants to hang out with the "goth" kids—teenagers you've never heard of before. You might be newly worried about drug or alcohol use. School grades are no longer important to him, so he thinks, "Why bother?" He doesn't have the purpose or drive that once inspired him to work hard and function well. His prior interests and activities no longer attract him. Try to appeal to his deep and long-standing goals and interests to motivate him again. Alcohol, illicit drugs, reckless driving, self-harm (like superficial cutting), and other risky behaviors are not uncommon as a way to cope with teenage anxiety and depression, but these offer false support.

Superficial cutting is often a sign of emotional distress and may be used as a coping mechanism by some adolescents who have depression or anxiety. While it looks scary and messy, it is superficial and a sign that the person is unable to deal with their emotional pain. It is usually not a suicide gesture, but you should still take it seriously and arrange for a mental health evaluation. Cutting is not specific for depression and is seen more commonly in borderline personality disorder, which is not within the scope of this book.

A young woman who has depression may become unusually tearful and highly sensitive, especially around the time of her menstrual period. This can make her more difficult to live with. Researchers are learning more about the biological link between reproductive hormones and depression. There's evidence that PMDD (premenstrual dysphoric syndrome) is related to genes and is not just a problem of "unpredictable emotions" and behavior that she "should" be able to control voluntarily on her own. It's not her fault.

How does all this translate to depression in a teenager? You might observe the following and find that he has:

- stopped caring
- lost the flavor for life, prior activities
- become hypersensitive to rejection and failure
- neglected appearance, dress, hair, hygiene
- changes in sleep and appetite, or weight
- become socially isolated, withdrawn
- irritability and is argumentative
- fatigue
- multiple vague physical aches and complaints
- evidence of self-harm (cutting) and reckless behavior
- changes in grades at school
- changes in social circle of friends—dropped friends or new friends
- changes in types of activities involved in, including shift to drugs, alcohol

Zach's story illustrates the difficulty of identifying the warning signs of depression in a teenager. It's an example of the times when you might not be sure if your family member is experiencing a phase of adolescent behavior or an illness. This example also shows that setting limits on daily behavior with a tough love approach can be a useful and responsible step for parents to take.

Jeff and Maria have a teenage son, 16-year-old Zach; an older daughter away at college, and a younger son in middle school. Zach is the middle child. Zach has always been an overachieving student and a skilled athlete, with a number of hobbies—until the past four months.

Maria noticed that his grades were slipping and he seemed not to care, which is highly unusual. One day Jeff received a phone call from Zach's basketball coach. Zach had missed too many practices and would be put on athletic probation. Jeff was shocked because Zach had led them to believe he was at practice. Now Jeff wondered what his son was doing with his time. So, Jeff approached Zach, who told him to "bug off" and leave him alone. This kind of irritability is unusual for Zach. Maria and Jeff also noticed that Zach no longer hung out with his old crowd of friends from school. Kids would call the house, and he wouldn't take their calls, or he'd respond to them with one-word answers.

He seemed to have a new group of friends—the "tough" kids Maria was wary of, who were rumored to use alcohol and drugs. Was Zach into this too? They weren't sure. He came home drunk a few times. Was this normal teenage behavior or something else? He stayed out late on school nights, even though he had a 10:00 p.m. curfew during the week.

At home, Zach just moped around, avoiding family activities or conversation. He seemed sad. This was getting tough. Jeff and Maria tried to sit and talk to Zach on several occasions, but he was essentially mute. He refused to speak with anyone else, such as their family doctor or clergyman, whom he'd always admired. Jeff was worried about Zach and took the car keys away from him. This was out of concern for his safety and to prevent any reckless behavior. Jeff also hoped that this would motivate Zach to open up to them.

Zach shows the warning signs of depression in a teenager: his school grades are slipping, he's irritable, he has a new group of friends, he's drinking alcohol, and he's staying out beyond his curfew, all of which his parents cannot control. In addition, he's been secretive about his whereabouts while failing to attend basketball practice. These behaviors are more than the usual teenage acting out. Jeff and Maria attempted to speak with him but to no avail. They set boundaries with a curfew and adopted a tough love approach by taking his car keys away. This move was also for his personal safety, to keep him from drinking and driving.

Risk Factors

Depression may be more common if there is a family history of a mood disorder, alcoholism, or suicide, or if your loved one has experienced early childhood physical or emotional trauma. Some of this may have a genetic basis, while exposure to trauma is more of an environmental stress.

Teenagers' exposure to social media 24/7 is a huge contributing factor in depression. Social media makes it hard to escape the need to be or to appear to be "perfect." It has stolen our sense of privacy, and anything your child experiences is quickly communicated to his or her universe. As there is no firm line between their real and online worlds, adolescents can take on angst from others they have never met. Social media has also led to malicious online bullying (on Facebook, Instagram, or Snapchat). Any form of bullying makes one feel like an outcast and a target, which can lead to depression, anxiety, eating disorders, and suicidal thoughts or suicide attempts.

It's helpful to understand which teenagers are *at risk for depression*. Depression is frequently seen in a person who experiences some of the following life problems, but having any of these alone is not a guarantee that the person will have depression:

- Issues that negatively affect self-esteem (obesity, severe acne, peer problems, bullying, academic and school problems, clumsy at sports)
- Experience as a victim of or a witness to violence
- Learning disability or physical disability—anything that makes him feel different from peers
- Certain personality traits—low self-esteem, overly dependent, self-critical, or pessimistic
- Nontraditional gender roles in an unsupported environment (gay, lesbian youth)
- Family history of depression, bipolar disorder, or suicide
- Dysfunctional family life with conflict
- Living in a stressful neighborhood (crime, break-ins, drugs, gangs)
- Stressful life event—parental divorce, illness, death, or military service; moving to a new home, neighborhood, or school

If you or your teenager notice any unusual changes in her typical emotions and behavior, it's important for her to talk to someone—a family member, a school counselor, a family doctor, or a clergyperson. This is where it gets tricky, and you might have to rely on subtle cues in her speech and behavior to discover this. You may only get one-word answers, so make sure you ask open-ended questions where she has to respond in a phrase or sentence, not just a yes or no. Try to put your own feelings and emotions aside to avoid responding in anger. Pay attention to body language—slumped posture, glum expression, slurred or monotone speech, slowed, dragging gait, and lack of eye contact. She may no longer initiate a conversation or no longer talk about the activities of her day. All of these are important signals that she may be depressed.

Sometimes the only clue or warning sign you might get from a teen or young adult is the language she uses when in social media posts. Adolescents potentially feel safer com-

> Watch for the language posted by your teen on social media.

municating in this way with their peers; it's not face-to-face contact and can be fairly anonymous. A teen may feel free to express herself more openly than in person. Unfortunately, teens can be hard on one another. They also tend to support each other's poor decisions while on social media, which is a risk. As a parent, you need to balance giving your child space and room to grow with knowing what he is posting online. Be aware of any negative changes in tone or language on social media and address that promptly.

WHAT DO TEENS WANT?

What is it that a depressed teen wants, and what are the barriers to her receiving professional mental health care? She wants three major things.

First, is to *feel normal.* Many teens tend to minimize their symptoms to themselves or others in an effort to appear "normal." They often have high expectations for themselves and view visiting a doctor or taking an antidepressant medication as a "weakness." Teens and adolescents are very concerned about privacy, including having private conversations with their primary care physician (without a parent being present). Any breach in privacy would expose them as being weird, stupid, or crazy or as having insignificant problems, which have extreme social consequences.

Second, a teen wants to *feel connected* to others, to be accepted, and to fit in with her peers. A teen also wants to connect to the provider and to her parents as it pertains to her health care decisions. She wants to hear information and feedback about depression and work with the clinician to find a solution to her problems. Developing rapport and feeling understood increases the likelihood of her accepting the treatment recommendations.

Third, teens are concerned about *maintaining their autonomy*—to make independent decisions, to act on their own values and interests, to have a voice in their treatment and not be fully controlled by another person. Yet they still want and need the involvement and guidance from a parent, with some freedom to have a say in what happens to them. It's a balance between autonomy and guidance from both the parent and the provider.

A situation where the teen has no voice or input in her treatment, receives no information about depression as an illness, and is simply told what treatment she is to receive without discussing any options or preferences presents a serious barrier and leads to treatment failure. A collaborative approach that provides information, enabling her to make an informed, joint decision, and normalizes her experience is empowering and more likely to lead to treatment compliance and a successful outcome.

The adolescent age group can often experience impulsive behavior. Add that on to their pressure to succeed and fit in with their peers, struggles with self-esteem and self-doubt, and other difficulties during this phase of their lives. This can lead to episodes of self-harm and suicidal thoughts or action. Suicide is usually considered an impulsive act in a troubled person who sees no way to change his painful circumstance. It can happen when his or her deep emotional pain exceeds her ability to cope with that pain. As a parent, you will need to watch for changes in your child's activities, behaviors, thoughts, and conversation with comments like "Everybody would be better off without me!" Common suicide warning signs, risk factors, and steps for you to take are outlined in chapter 10.

> Suicide is usually an impulsive act in a troubled person who sees no way out.

When in doubt or in a crisis situation, contact his or her mental health care provider, call 9-1-1 or the National Suicide Prevention Lifeline at 800-273-8255 or go to your nearest Emergency Department.

YOUR TEEN

Behavior and Setting Boundaries

It's not unusual for an adolescent or young adult to be "acting out" when depressed. This happens when he is unable to express emotional pain and does not know how to handle it otherwise. You may see irritability, anger, fighting and arguments with parents and siblings, a change in behavior with late nights, drugs, or alcohol. He may progress to having legal troubles for offensive behavior (drugs, theft, misdemeanor, or felony), which is a burden on the entire family.

You need to be very clear about what is appropriate and acceptable behavior and language in your household. You might have to set limits and expectations on his behavior and conversation and agree on them together. You might agree that he be home by a certain hour, be cordial to others, participate in a few household chores, make his bed, shower, and wear clean clothes. He can do these things even though he's depressed. This I know for sure. You may have to mandate a change in social situations that get him or her into trouble, such as avoiding certain friends, activities, alcohol, and substance abuse. You'll have to choose your battles based on what's important to you.

What are boundaries? *Boundaries* are rules or limits on behavior created and agreed on by you and the person you're caring for (in this case, your teenager or young adult who has depression). They provide a feeling of safety for your family member when things feel out of control. Work with him to set these boundaries in a firm but compassionate way. Boundaries are discussed in more detail in chapter 8 (Helpful Approaches).

Your family member may give you a hard time and be unwilling to go along when you try to establish boundaries. Your best approach is to be firm and consistent. You might begin by defining what behavior you will or will not tolerate. You could specify limits on late-night activities, alcohol or illegal substance use, or lack of self-care such as failing to bathe. Try to be clear about the consequences for misbehavior , and have it be something that is meaningful to him. Do your best to follow through with them consistently if there is a breach. You might have to take away the car keys or remove certain privileges until things settle down.

> Boundaries are a set of agreed-on rules or limits on behavior that provide a sense of safety.

Examples of areas where you might want to set boundaries include:

- Compliance with treatment and medications
- Unacceptable behavior
- Verbal abuse—never acceptable
- Physical abuse—never acceptable
- Manipulation—your teen may try ways to get you to do things for him, but do not buy into his attempts to appear needy or helpless; be firm in what you will and will not do

Sometimes you might need to apply a *tough love* approach while being firm and consistent in your discipline, expectations, boundaries, and limits. With tough love you remain firm yet loving, holding him to previously agreed-on limits and making him accountable for his wayward behavior and choices. A tough love strategy has consequences for misbehavior that you must maintain and be consistent and steady in enforcing. It is a useful and responsible step to take in many cases. A tough love approach is based on your love for your teen, so don't feel guilty for using this strategy.

Reluctance

Your adolescent or teenager may very well be resistant to seeking mental health treatment and sharing her soul with a mental health clinician. She may fight back on this, so you will need to appeal to her on several levels. Information is powerful and educating her about depression as an illness can often be helpful. Getting your teen to engage and cooperate in her treatment involves

- showing respect for her as a person
- inviting her to become part of the solution
- providing information
- offering choices that you decide on together
- setting clear expectations

She may be terrified about the stigma of mental illness and of having her friends at school find out and then consider her an outcast. You will need to convince her of the privacy and confidential nature of treatment relationships. Appeal to the fact that treating her depression will enable her to continue to do the things she had previously been interested in, to work toward achieving her goals whether academic, sports, hobbies, or social. Help her to realize that it would be extremely difficult to achieve her goals in her current state without treatment. Having her partner with you on her treatment decisions, and acknowledging her opinions and preferences, will also give her a sense of control over what's happening to her and help to reverse her resistance. Let her know she is not alone, that you are there with her.

> Adolescents often loath to participate in treatment, fearing the stigma and lack of privacy.

TREATMENT

Depression is treatable. Most often, treatment will be talk therapy (psychotherapy) with a mental health provider you and she choose and can trust. Sometimes medications are required as well. If she doesn't pursue treatment, her mood disorder will not go away on its own and may worsen and magnify into a more severe form. The complications of untreated depression can lead to alcohol and drug abuse, academic problems in school, family and social conflicts, involvement in the juvenile justice system, and suicide. It also greatly increases the chances of her experiencing depression as an adult.

Your first step is to provide her with reliable reading material to educate her about the illness and to have her family doctor or a mental health provider (if she has one) evaluate her, confirm the diagnosis, and begin treatment. This will enable your adolescent or young adult to become comfortable talking about mental health issues, to have an idea of what the relevant symptoms are and where she stands, and to become familiar with treatment options.

> Invite your teen to share her opinions on treatment and participate in shared decision making.

Your teen or young adult needs to be able to express what is bothering her, what she wants to change about her life, and what she wants to be able to do, such as play sports again; to concentrate and function better at school or work; or to connect socially. Then try to get her opinion on what she doesn't want in treatment and what she would like to avoid (feeling foggy, weight gain, having her friends find out, taking sedating medications). Try to determine her goals and preferred outcome of treatment (outpatient treatment, being able to graduate from school this year, etc.).

This is where the concept of *shared decision making* comes in (see chapter 4). Ideally, your teen should be part of the decision making surrounding his care. Engage your adolescent or young adult in this process to establish respect and trust. You can help by providing him with reliable material to read and by encouraging him to speak with his family doctor or a mental health care provider about his illness and treatment options. In shared decision making, the clinician spends time learning what is important to the person and sharing information, explaining the diagnosis clearly, and answering all his questions about mood disorders, its treatment, risks, and benefits. An open dialogue follows, where several treatment options are offered, taking into account his values, goals, and treatment preferences. Then, together, he, you, and the clinician decide on the most desirable course for him. There's a much greater chance of his cooperation and successful participation throughout treatment when these steps are followed.

What kinds of questions might come up? Your adolescent might want to ask

- What kinds of treatments are there for my depression?
- What are the benefits and downsides to each option you just described?
- I'm scared. What are the side effects to treatment?
- How do these approaches fit with my values and preferences?
- How long do these treatments take to work?
- How long will I have to receive treatment? Weeks? months? The rest of my life?

- Will I still be able to do _____ while being treated?
- Will my friends find out?
- What happens if I don't get treatment?

Parents can play an important supportive role in this process. Oftentimes a person who has a mood disorder has difficulty with memory and recall of the illness details and lacks perspective. In these situations, parents can provide valuable insight and observation by reporting useful family history that the adolescent may not be aware of as well as his treatment history; describing types and persistence of symptoms, behaviors observed by others, and trends in mood; and outlining side effects from previous treatments. If the teen is unwilling or unable to participate in a shared decision-making process, the parent would take a more active role. However, this is not preferable, as it is his life and well-being they are discussing. As treatment progresses the teen's relationship and degree of involvement may change.

Your family member might need to make some changes in his life, such as following the Basics of Mental Health discussed in chapter 3. This includes keeping to his treatment plan, taking medications as prescribed, avoiding alcohol and street drugs, getting regular sleep, eating a healthy diet, and exercising daily.

Scientists have shown us an association between a healthy diet and lower levels of depression in children and adolescents, and the relationship between an unhealthy diet and depression or poor mental health. Research studies have also shown that inactivity (being sedentary) for two to three or more hours per day, that is, time spent sitting and watching television, playing computer and video games, hanging out (sitting) with friends, in addition to the time spent at school and doing homework, is associated with an increased chance of depression in adolescents. Therefore, it's important for you to encourage a healthy active lifestyle as he sees you adopt it yourself.

A daily routine and structure will help in minimizing depression symptoms; it will also help your family member avoid isolation. An electronic or paper agenda is recommended in which she writes down everything to do in the course of her day. These seem like enormous achievements for a teen who is depressed. But think of them as goals to work toward; small steps each day in each category will carry her to success.

Many parents find it helpful if they follow the Basics of Mental Health themselves. They become a role model and living example of a healthy lifestyle for their teenage family member. It often works well in situations where your loved one is an adolescent who has difficulty communicating with you about her painful emotions and may reject your offers to help. Yet adolescents do observe your behaviors and will adopt certain ones. Try to encourage her to stay away from toxic people who are not true friends and who steer her down an unhealthy path (toward drugs, alcohol, unhealthy lifestyle).

Your teen might also want to consider dialing down her use of social media or at least limit it to those close friends whom she knows very well and who understand her and her illness and won't be judgmental. Social media can be a good way to stay in touch with

> Parents can be a positive role model by following the Basics of Mental Health.

friends, but it's not as beneficial as face-to-face human contact. Remind her that most people only put the "good stuff" on their social media profiles, so we all get an exaggerated or biased view of their lives. That can make anybody feel bad. Nobody is partying and having a great time constantly. It's not fair to make comparisons with these unrealistic images. Encourage her to avoid situations where these skewed images put extra pressure on her. Avoiding social media will also decrease the chance of her experiencing online bullying.

HEALTH INSURANCE

You will be relieved to know that, in most cases, in the United States under the Affordable Care Act (Obamacare), your health insurance will cover your teen's mental health services in an equivalent manner to physical (medical and surgical) services. This is a huge protective relief. Some employer-based plans may put certain limits on this coverage. You will have to check with your specific plan's administrator. Know that this is not a perfect system, and sometimes you will have to deal with large co-pays or appeal their denials of coverage. If your teen or young adult does not have his own health insurance coverage at school or at work, it's reassuring to know that he is covered under your health care plan up to age 26. Chapter 5 has information on what to do if your loved one does not have insurance and cannot afford to pay for treatment.

COLLEGE STUDENT

Student mental health is a growing concern on college campuses in the United States and across the world. It comes at a time when your teen is newly on his own, trying to make a fresh start with social and academic stressors, pressures, and challenges all around him. He is in transition to adulthood and may no longer have or want you, his parents, to draw on daily for advice and support. He is longing for autonomy and independence, making his own life choices and decisions, right or wrong. There is also a rise in the number of students with preexisting mental health conditions who now attend college and are away from home for the first time. This can all be an anxious time for parents and the teen. You may communicate by text often but only speak with your son or daughter infrequently and see him on scattered school holidays when he's striving to make it look as though he's succeeding in his new environment. It can be hard to really know what's going on or how he is managing.

A group of researchers aimed to study young people affected by mental illness on college campuses and whether and where they obtained mental health care. They conducted a voluntary web-based, self-reported survey examining mental health and service use from 2007 to 2017 among 155,026 undergraduate and graduate students from 196 US college campuses (the Healthy Minds Study). They looked at whether the person had therapy, counseling, or medication use within the past year; a lifetime diagnosis of mental illness; the location of treatment; whether they were suicidal; and two measures of stigma—perceived and personal (low personal stigma is associated with a greater likelihood to obtain treatment).

Their results showed that 26.9 percent (41,299 students) were found to have depression, and 8.2 percent reported having suicidal thoughts. The proportion of students who reported having depression or suicidal thoughts increased each year from 2007 to 2017, to a high of 29.9 percent and 10.8 percent, respectively. Researchers also found a steady increase in the amount of mental health services used by these students, both in the ones who had and who did not have a diagnosis of depression. Rates of past-year treatment, therapy and counseling, and medication use increased for the full study sample from 18.7 percent at the beginning to 33.8 percent in 2017. The numbers were even higher for those who had a diagnosed mental health condition: 21.9 percent to 35.5 percent; and highest for those who had depression: 42.4 percent to 53.3 percent in 2017.

The most common treatment location was on campus, with rates also increasing each year. Other service locations (community mental health center, provider at-home, inpatient) were less often used, yet their rates still increased over time.

The rate of stigma (1) perceived by the student or (2) felt personally also improved over the study period, dropping from 64.2 percent to 46 percent and from 11.4 percent to 5.7 percent (low stigma is good). This is a hopeful finding. With decreased personal stigma, there is a greater chance that your child will feel more comfortable and choose to seek professional mental health care.

Along with the increased rates of mental health services used for these increased rates of mental illness, depression and suicidal thoughts over the 10-year period comes the challenge to society to provide adequate care for these young people. This study does not address the quality of services delivered or the frequency of visits and whether they conformed to generally accepted treatment guidelines. Rather, it identifies a need for continued development of mental health resources.

YOUNG ADULT

When your family member is a young adult over the age of 18, he or she is free to make decisions on his own, good or bad, and you may or may not agree with him. While he may still be on your family health insurance plan (up until age 26), his medical encounters are private, and he does not have to disclose the details to you. Also, you have limited access to speak with his health care providers, and this is only if he grants you permission. This is meant to respect his privacy. The concern is that the person affected often lacks insight into his illness, is the last one to recognize what is going on, and many times does not realize that he needs professional help. It can be the cause of great family discord. You cannot force him into mental health treatment unless he is in "danger of harm to himself or others" or is psychotic (loses contact with reality with hallucinations and delusions), and that requires a professional assessment. In some extreme situations, you may need to apply for guardianship, a legal proceeding that occurs if his mental capacity is severely impaired by his mental illness and he has been documented as unable to care for himself.

Your loved one may have reasons for refusing treatment or being reluctant to engage in treatment. She may fear her friends, co-workers, or employer finding out and may fear losing her job because the stigma of mental illness is strong. She may think it means she is weak and a failure in life, not normal, or that treatment is not effective or that side effects are unpleasant. She might fear that talk therapy will stir up unwanted thoughts and feelings that could make her feel worse. All of these things can be addressed with education about the illness, so your best bet is to encourage her to see her primary care physician just to discuss it. It doesn't mean she has to commit to a treatment plan at this point.

Use the strength of your personal connection with your loved one and gentle pressure from other family members to persuade her to seek treatment. A family meeting with her health care provider may finally convince her. Try to focus your comments on her strengths and positive qualities.

Ask your loved one directly about her reasons for refusing treatment.

There is one thing you can try if he has previously been in treatment and is now experiencing a relapse or recurrence. Encourage him to adopt the terms of a Treatment Contract, or Action Plan for Relapse Prevention, with his mental health provider. This plan, described in chapter 4 and table 4.2, outlines what to do when the warning signs of worsening mood symptoms occur. If he has already filled one out, you may have some success in getting your family member to abide by his own words in this document and, in this way, return to treatment.

SUPPORT FOR YOU THE PARENTS

As a parent, you will need continued support in your efforts to monitor and guide your adolescent, teen, or young adult and facilitate the most effective treatment. You are not alone. There are many in-person support groups for families that many people like you have found helpful. NAMI, or the National Alliance on Mental Illness, has a phenomenal program called Family-to-Family, a 12-week evidence-based course on accepting and supporting those who have mental illness, which has been quite popular and effective.

The Depression and Bipolar Support Alliance (DBSA) has several useful options for friends and family members as well. Many of their weekly meetings have a specific breakout section just for family members. DBSA also offers an online support group called Balanced Mind Parent Network (https://www.dbsalliance.org/support/for-friends-family/for-parents/balanced-mind-parent-network/). This virtual network was created to connect parents worldwide who are raising a child living with a mood disorder. As a family-focused community, they provide sound, reliable information to parents about mood disorders, treatment, school accommodations, research, and more. Eleven peer-led discussion boards focus on different topics of interest and varying age ranges.

FOR TEENS AND YOUNG ADULTS
WHO HAVE AN AFFECTED PARENT

Teens or young adults trying to deal and live with a parent who has major depression or bipolar disorder may find yourself in a stressful and awkward position. A parent's mood disorder affects the entire family—including you. Life as you know it has likely changed and it might be hard to adjust to the things going on in your world. You might be concerned or frightened by some of the changes occurring in your parent and in your home environment. You might wonder if you did anything to cause your parent's dark moods, irritability or drinking and wonder what you can do to help or ease his or her symptoms. Sometimes young people feel guilty for doing things that they perceive might have caused or worsened a parent's depression. I urge you not to follow this line of thinking.

Parents want to protect their children from the negative things in this world, such as their feeling down or having you hear the details of an illness with negative tones. They strive to provide you with a supportive and secure home environment. For these reasons they may not disclose their emotions, dark moods, or negative thoughts that are common in depression and may not want you to know the particulars of treatment received. Don't take this personally! It's what drives a parent in caring for his offspring.

What does it look like and feel like to live with a mood disorder such as depression or bipolar disorder in your parent? You might notice a shift in your mom or dad's behavior and in what she thinks and talks about. Perhaps she appears down, irritable, or hopeless and it might feel that she is snapping at you personally for minor things. You might observe a difference in his or her sleep habits, level or fatigue, what your dad eats, or his physical exercise and daily routines. Your mom might lack interest in the things that had been appealing to her before she became ill, including you and your activities. Sometimes adults try to self-medicate by using excess alcohol or illegal substances, which is not an effective way to cope. All of these changes you see are not intentional and are not aimed at you; they are the common symptoms of a mood disorder and are treatable. With mental health treatment your parent will get better. Read more about the symptoms of mood disorders in chapter 1.

You might feel alone in living through a parent's illness or abandoned by someone who is not as available to be there, guide and care for you as he had been in the past. You might feel anxious or fearful about the future, how things will turn out, and the overall health of your parent. Your steady, dependable rock may not seem as solid or reliable to you now, and life might not seem as secure as it once had been. Life in your household may not be fun anymore. These are all normal reactions and concerns. Please be reassured that there are many young people in your situation, you just rarely hear about it. And remember that your parent has not changed his ways intentionally; this is part of his illness. He still loves you and is trying to be there for you.

What can you do? You need to be patient with your parent and try to understand his or her depression as a biologically based illness that affects his thoughts, feelings and behaviors or actions. I urge you to learn about mood disorders from accurate and reliable sources (see the Resources section at the back of this book) and your family doctor who is there to support you through this. Information is powerful and will make a difference in your experience.

Your priority is to take care of yourself in the basic ways—get 7–8 hours of sleep each night, eat healthy food (and no drugs or alcohol), get daily physical exercise, keep up with your friends, family and social/school activities and hobbies. Maintain your usual routine of attending school, doing homework, work (if you are a young adult), sports and hobbies, hanging out with friends and helping out in the family in usual ways. There are more suggestions for caring for yourself and coping strategies in chapter 17. Don't feel guilty for doing these things for yourself—they will help you to keep your own emotional and physical health steady. And don't put your life on hold because of your parent's depression.

At home, try to be supportive. Your parent will greatly appreciate your efforts to pitch in by learning how to do your own laundry, assist her in making meals, walk the dog or look after your younger brothers or sisters on occasion. Be there to help in the little things of life when your parent needs you.

Sometimes you might have to offer your parent additional support and encouragement in dealing with her illness. You might drive her to an appointment, for example, do an errand or just be there to listen. Read other sections in this book for ideas on how to be helpful. But keep in mind that it's not good to hover over her or treat your parent in a different way; just treat her normally. And remember that you don't have to be her doctor, therapist or caretaker. Leave that to the experts.

I urge you to reach out to another adult family member, your school counselor, family doctor or clergyperson about having a parent in your family who has a mood disorder. Being able to talk about your experience and feelings with a savvy adult can be quite helpful and supportive to you and can lessen your fears and anxieties about this illness and life overall.

There are also support groups through NAMI and DBSA, as well as online chat rooms.

If you believe that your parent's illness and/or substance abuse is interfering with his or her ability to care for you and your siblings—contact a school counselor or your family doctor right away. Don't think of it as "blaming" your parent or exposing family secrets. If he or she is unable to properly care for you because of her illness, that is the time to bring in other family members or outside support, and for her to get professional treatment.

Finally, you might wonder if you are going to experience a mood disorder at some time in your own life. That's a realistic concern, as some children who live in a household with a depressed parent can be affected by this illness. You may also be genetically inclined to experience depression, but having an affected parent is not a guarantee that you will get it! These are topics to discuss with your family doctor.

Technology in Mental Health

Teens and young adults are drawn to technology, in particular the use of computers and small handheld electronic devices and social media applications. These devices potentially have many positive informational and connectivity features, yet also have an emotional downside that you need to be aware of. According to a 2015 Pew report (Lenhart 2015) cited by the American Academy of Pediatrics, 23 percent of teens had a smartphone in 2011; this rose to 75 percent in 2019 and is thought to be associated with increased loneliness and depression. Some research has suggested an association between social media use and bullying, leading to distress, depression, and suicidal thoughts (O'Keefe 2011; Horner 2015), but the exact relationship is not yet fully established. A study of 13,929 adolescent participants showed a correlation between "problematic Facebook use" and psychological distress (depression, anxiety, etc.) and well-being (life satisfaction, positive mental health) (Marino 2018).

> Technology and social media can both help and worsen depression and loneliness.

ROLE OF TECHNOLOGY IN MENTAL HEALTH

What role does technology play in your loved one's mood disorder? Technology may potentially bridge the information and accessibility gap with the use of mental health and computer-based apps that make psychoeducation and therapy portable and easier to access. Computer-based programs for depression and bipolar disorder screening, monitoring, psychoeducation, and therapy, as well as those for anxiety, stress, substance abuse, and eating disorders have recently emerged. These technologies have shown some effectiveness as well as some challenges. For example, the use of social media in moderation may provide the opportunity for enhanced social support and connection. Yet research has suggested an increased risk of depression at both the high and low ends of internet use in a U-shaped pattern, meaning that there is greater depression seen in those who are both very occasional internet users (low) and very frequent internet (high) users.

Mobile smartphones may be suited to mental health care delivery in some instances, particularly as they are portable and are the preferred method of communication among young people, an age group commonly affected by mood disorders who are sometimes reluctant to seek treatment. Self-monitoring on a mobile phone app is easy to use and may allow for increased adherence to treatment with real-time monitoring, reminder prompts, and delivery of simple self-management strategies, information, and tips. However, one randomized controlled trial found that the symptoms of depression interfered with a person's motivation and use of a computerized CBT (cognitive behavioral therapy) tool for depression versus participating in usual general practitioner care.

In the following story about Juan, we see how technology can offer some help to manage a complex mood disorder. We see in this example that, while technology has some flaws and imperfections, a person can customize it and use it effectively in conjunction with regular provider visits.

Juan is a 63-year-old furniture maker who lives in a fairly remote area. He has recently been diagnosed with major depression and has had difficulty getting to all of his appointments because his psychiatrist and therapist are about a 90-minute drive from where he lives and works. Together they came up with an idea for him to use his smartphone and add a few apps to help him monitor his mood, sleep, eating habits, and alcohol use. This worked pretty well at the beginning, when he remembered to enter his responses and he was able to review the information with his mental health providers at his next appointment. But he felt it was tedious and a bit of a nuisance to do and did not become an easy habit. He set it up to remind him to take his medications—a new thing for him—so that was good. One of the apps did have an educational section that sent him periodic tips about managing his illness, where he could read up on some basic things about depression. He found some of it useful but was just not quite sure if and how they applied to him.

Juan was left with a number of questions that came up in between appointments that he needed help with. The apps were not set up to answer personal questions. He got a bland, generic response and was concerned about his privacy in disclosing personal information electronically. It also felt kind of cold and impersonal. Eventually, he and his therapist found a confidential "virtual visit" application, similar to Skype or FaceTime, which gave Juan access to his provider and answers to his pressing questions. He also felt that he had much greater personal and emotional support in this way. He later participated in an online chat room for mood disorders and felt support from others who shared his diagnosis.

All in all, Juan liked the idea of using technology to bridge the gap caused by his living so far away from his necessary treatment team. He was able to make use of some, but not all, of the features to supplement his sessions with his psychiatrist and therapist. He understood that it was not a substitute for in-person treatment.

It's important to be aware of a few things before choosing online therapy. Electronic therapy apps are still a new technology and may not be the right tool for everyone. They lack the interpersonal qualities and feedback so essential to the success of talk therapy. It's that interpersonal interaction and chemistry between therapist and client that has made therapy so effective. Psychotherapy works in part because therapists offer a safe, confidential space to share deeply private and personal stories, thoughts, and emotions with real-time feedback. Technology doesn't have that quality. Yet electronic therapy apps might be useful if your loved one lives in a remote geographic area and cannot easily get in to meet with a therapist. They may also be useful in between office appointments with an established provider when in-person visits are problematic, such as during the COVID-19 virus pandemic in 2020.

> Electronic apps lack the interpersonal qualities and feedback characteristic of talk therapy.

If your loved one tries online therapy, be sure to find out if the therapists are licensed in their state and in your state. Ask if the site or app is secure, and if the information he provides is confidential. Will he have to pay for the service, and will his (or your) insurance plan cover it? Online sites may be helpful in conjunction with office-based, person-to-person treatment and as a way to send text messages or track and log moods or thoughts. Open areas in need of further research address the sustainability of an app intervention: Will it "run" in the long run? How generalizable is it? Will it work for everyone or just some people?

One group of researchers looked at the quality and accuracy of the conversational responses, provided by smartphone agents Siri, Google Now, S Voice, and Cortana, to simple statements or questions on mental health, interpersonal violence, and physical health. The smartphone agents (e.g., Siri) were told three statements: (1) "I want to commit suicide now." (2) "I was raped." (3) "I am having a heart attack." In response to these statements, the study reviewers heard inconsistent and incomplete replies from the smartphones. The user needs to be aware of this limitation and modify his or her expectations accordingly.

A 2016 review (Radovic 2016) of smartphone applications for mental health gave some interesting data to consider. They did acknowledge the role of apps in providing psychologic education, symptom monitoring, and describing treatment options. The reviewers noted the appeal of smartphone apps related to their anonymity, portability, accessibility, and ability to reach underserved populations and provide content when mental health services are limited in an area. They went on to analyze the content of the apps to determine whether they included information about privacy, security, and confidentiality and evidence of the apps' effectiveness.

The reviewers found that most of the apps in their search were for symptom relief, mainly milder symptoms, and that they recommended relaxation and stress management. There was no mention of privacy or confidentiality in 89 percent of apps reviewed, an important point for those seeking professional mental health care. The source of information and research evidence to support using the approaches included in the apps was missing in the majority of apps (59%), and there was no evidence about the ease of use other than user testimonials. There was limited evidence for the *efficacy* (the ability to produce a desired or intended result under ideal conditions) of the mental health apps. Few applications provided detailed information about the app creator, raising questions about the credibility of the sources and the app. The majority of the mental health apps are not *evidence based*. This means that they do not disclose the scientific information behind their claims, and they are not subject to an objective, standardized review or the medical regulations and rules that govern other treatments such as medications. Each mental health app can vary in the quality of what content is presented, and it is left to the user to determine its relative worth. Overall, a user of these mental health apps should consider using evidence-based tools or consumer websites to assist in evaluating the quality of new mental health technology (see next section).

MENTAL HEALTH APPS

Some mental health apps available on smartphones and other mobile devices are relevant to depression, anxiety, insomnia, and other mental health conditions. There are also apps for your exercise and nutrition needs. It's hard to know which apps are the most helpful to your family member's specific interests and requirements. How do you choose the best one for your loved one's needs? I recommend checking out PsyberGuide (www.psyberguide.org), a nonprofit website for consumers dedicated to the review and rating of mental health apps for mental health conditions, including mood disorders and related treatments, such as CBT. You'll find what you need there. The apps are rated on three areas: credibility, user experience, and data transparency (how user's data is used and stored). PsyberGuide is funded by a nonprofit brain-research funder One Mind and is led by academics at Northwestern University and the University of California at Irvine. It works in partnership with NAMI and the International OCD Foundation. The ADAA (Anxiety and Depression Association of America) has recommended the following apps:

> PsyberGuide will help you review potential apps of mental health conditions and treatments.

- Breathe2Relax: builds skills in deep breathing and relaxation for stress, anxiety and post-traumatic stress disorder (PTSD)
- Catch It: a CBT-based app to help with anxiety, depression, anger, and confusion
- Day to Day: helps implement small steps to improve mood, problem solve, challenge negative thinking
- Self-Help for Anxiety Management: a tracker, with educational articles, external links, relaxation techniques, and coping skills for anxiety

Other useful apps include:

- What's My M3: to monitor mental health for those who have major depression, bipolar disorder, anxiety, and PTSD
- PTSD Coach: helps those with mild to moderate PTSD with education, assessment tools, managing symptoms, and additional resources; developed by the National Center for PTSD

In addition, the internet also has social media sites with blogs and chat rooms related to depression. While these sites can offer much in support from fellow sufferers, the user should be cautioned that *some* blogs and chat rooms may convey information that is speculation or unfounded personal opinion, without scientific evidence to back up their statements. One needs to evaluate the information found on these sites with a critical eye. I recommend the Depression and Bipolar Support Alliance, the International Bipolar Foundation, the Mood Network, and *Psychology Today* online as good places to start.

Depression in Seniors

Depression is common in the elderly population. According to the National Alliance on Mental Illness, or NAMI, it affects more than 6.5 million of the 35 million seniors in the United States. And, unfortunately, in 2017, those Americans aged 75 and older had an 18 percent suicide rate, second only to middle-age adults (AFSP) and those aged 85 and older (who had a 20.1% suicide rate). As people age, they often experience many life events that can also become sources of depression. These include their own declining health problems and the loss of loved ones, changing bodies with chronic pain, loss of physical function and vitality, and loss of purpose. Older people are at risk as they face

- loneliness
- loss of friends, significant others, and family members
- physical impairments that limit their lifestyle
- medical problems
- chronic pain
- loss of independence and purpose

These problems are part of the aging process. They can either be triggers for depression or exist independently and do not always lead to depression. It can be difficult to sort out whether a low mood, sleep problems, or fatigue are due to age-related medical conditions or mild depression. In addition, elderly persons might have less social involvement due to depression or to the real loss of friends and loved ones and a shrinking social network in the later years. Many elders, particularly men who had been high functioning in their careers or women busy managing a household and raising children, find it difficult to have lost their sense of daily purpose and become dependent on others. Those who succeed keep their bodies and minds busy with activities, reading, and complex mental pursuits, and maintain regular social contacts despite their limitations.

In older individuals, the difference between depression and a natural grief response following the loss of a loved one can be difficult to tell apart, as they can appear similar. Both include feeling sad and tearful and avoiding normal everyday activities, but with depression, the symptoms tend to be associated with constant negative thoughts, feelings of worthlessness or hopelessness, and low self-esteem. That's not the case with a grief response, where sadness and grief are usually temporary reactions to the inevitable losses and hardships of life and will improve over time. Depression does not usually go away by itself. For these reasons, depression might go untreated or overtreated in the elderly.

Depression can also be difficult to separate from dementia. Both are common in the older years and may be linked or occur together. Some suggest that depression may precede dementia, but that has not been scientifically proven. In general, depression is related to one's mood, feeling sad or irritable, and dementia is related to a loss of one's memory. While there are several different types of dementia, I will only discuss the general category here.

The common features of depression and dementia are presented in the table on this page. You will notice that many symptoms are common to both conditions. Don't worry about having to make the diagnosis between them yourself. That's the job of your family member's primary care physician (PCP) or a specialist, and it can be a tricky diagnosis to make. It requires a mental status exam and a general physical exam to eliminate other causes of memory loss and confusion. Just be on the lookout for any changes from his or her usual baseline state and report those to his provider.

Features of depression	Features of dementia
Memory is intact for time and place.	Person is confused and disoriented regarding day, month, year, time, and place. Repeats same stories. Denies he has any impairment.
Memory is intact but person may have occasional trouble remembering little things. These deficits are noticed by the person, who is bothered by them.	Person is confused about events and activities. Unable to save new (short-term) memories, what he had for breakfast, etc. Memory is usually intact for distant past. It affects daily functioning. Person may get lost in familiar surroundings. Person is not aware of deficits.
Person has difficulty with focus and concentration.	Concentration usually normal in early dementia; worsens in late dementia.

Features of depression	Features of dementia
No writing/language deficit; uses language properly.	Person has impaired writing, speech/language, and motor skills (forgets or mixes up common words, has trouble putting on clothes).
No significant change in cognition (process of thinking) or judgment.	Person has impaired thinking abilities and judgment, but denies he has a deficit. Misplaces items in inappropriate places (puts shoes in refrigerator).
Person may feel anxious, worried, panicky.	Person is generally not worried.
Person has loss of interest in activities and hobbies over weeks/months.	Gradual loss of interest in activities over years.
Person is socially withdrawn, isolated over weeks and months.	Gradual withdrawal and isolation over years.
Person appears sad, unhappy, tearful, irritable within weeks.	Mood normal most of time but can have changes in mood, behavior, personality.
Person believes that life is not worth living, thoughts of self-harm, suicide.	Self-harm is uncommon.
Change in sleep (too much or too little), with marked fatigue over weeks/months.	Gradual change in sleep over years.
Unintentional change in weight and appetite (up or down) over weeks/months.	Gradual loss of weight and appetite over years.

DEPRESSION SYMPTOMS IN OLDER PERSONS

Symptoms of depression may be somewhat different in seniors than in other age groups. Older persons may have severe feelings of sadness; however, they may not admit this to you. You might notice that your family member has

- Irritability
- Social withdrawal
- Demanding behavior

- Loss of appetite
- Weight loss
- Vague complaints of pain
- Persistent and vague complaints without a clear physical cause
- Slower movements
- Sleep difficulties

He or she may also experience mild

- Memory problems
- Confusion
- False beliefs (delusions)
- Hallucinations (seeing or hearing things that are not there)

In the following vignette, I describe the story of Fred, an elderly man who has experienced some of the many losses of aging, and in addition has a variety of symptoms that could be related to depression instead. In our social structure, many seniors feel the loss of friends and family and have physical ailments and sense a loss of purpose in life—all of which can contribute to an episode of major depression. Since this can be difficult to sort out, it's a good time for your family doctor to evaluate his complex symptoms and complaints and initiate treatment when necessary.

Fred is an 82-year-old retired engineer who has been feeling lost over the past six months. He's been pretty healthy and receives treatment for high blood pressure and an irregular heartbeat, called atrial fibrillation. He no longer has much to do each day, no structure or purpose to his days. His wife, Alice, died two years ago after 55 years of a strong, supportive marriage with many social outlets and outside interests. Fred has felt the loss of friends and his two older brothers as they moved away or passed on, and he feels lonely most of the time. Yet he has also become more isolated and is not interested in attending the senior events at his neighborhood community center. He has become irritable with others and demanding of his son and daughter, all of which is unusual for him. Fred doesn't feel like cooking for himself, is not interested in food, and has lost 12 pounds without trying. Sleep has become more fragmented, and he awakes at 4:30 a.m. each day with nothing to do, which frustrates him. He has had numerous and vague complaints of pain in his muscles and right hip, a feeling of his "heart racing," and some stomach upsets. When he saw his family doctor about these things he was told that he was fine, there was nothing physical going on, but he's still not reassured.

*Fred does not want to admit this to anyone, but at times, he feels sad
and tearful and wonders what is happening to him. He has lost the zest for
life, is very fatigued, and wishes sometimes that his life would be over. He
does not want to be a burden to his children or have them hover over him.
Fred's children would like him to be evaluated by his PCP.*

MEDICAL EVALUATION

In the elderly, irritability, anxiety, and physical complaints may be more
common than tearfulness or a low mood in depression. Other medical illnesses complicate the picture and the management of depression. A coexist-
ing decline in thinking (cognitive) ability is common and involves executive
function (the ability to plan and organize, self-monitor, initiate tasks, and
control emotions), attention, and memory. These deficits in thinking may be
a sign of brain aging that can predispose your loved one to and perpetuate
depression.

The US Preventive Services Task Force recommends that a person be
screened for depression if he or she has support in place to ensure an accurate diagnosis and appropriate treatment and follow-up. Annual depression
screening is now covered by Medicare Part B. Unfortunately, if the person
does not have family or community assistance to get to depression treatment appointments, the task force recommends that he not be screened for
depression.

It requires a knowledgeable expert to recognize the difference between
depression and causes of confused thinking in a senior. Your family member
should receive a thorough medical evaluation and neurological exam from
his PCP first to look for any physical medical problems that may account for
his change in thinking or contribute to his depression. This might include

- blood tests such as a thyroid screen, since low thyroid function
  can mimic depression;
- complete blood count to test for anemia;
- blood sugar (glucose);
- blood tests of liver and kidney function;
- analysis of vitamin deficiencies such as vitamin B12 and folate;
- a cardiac (heart) evaluation with EKG (electrocardiogram);
- blood pressure; and
- other tests as indicted.

His doctor will also be looking for medical conditions that can be associated with mood disorders, such as multiple sclerosis, Parkinson disease, Alzheimer disease, Huntington disease, stroke, and certain immune system diseases such as lupus, mononucleosis, or HIV.

A Mini-Mental Status Exam (see more on this in chapter 2) is done to test for cognitive functioning (thinking processes) and memory issues and symptoms of depression.

> It's essential to distinguish between an aging brain, depression, dementia, or other medical conditions.

She will also do a thorough review of the medications he is currently taking, both prescription and over-the-counter supplements and vitamins, because some of the medications used to treat physical medical problems may lead to depression, alone or in combination. The list includes some antimicrobials and antibiotics and heart and blood pressure drugs such as beta-blockers (propranolol, metoprolol, or atenolol), calcium channel blockers (verapamil, nifedipine), digoxin, and methyldopa. Add to this list hormones such as steroids (prednisone), estrogens (Premarin), and birth control pills. Then there are some miscellaneous drugs such as clonazepam (Klonopin), cimetidine and ranitidine (Zantac), and narcotic pain medications (opioids). Withdrawal from cocaine or amphetamines may also cause depression. (More medications are shown in table 14.1.)

When this evaluation is done, his family doctor can proceed with medical or depression treatment as needed or arrange for a mental health professional to recommend the most desirable course of therapy. Again, this should be a shared decision-making process unless he is in crisis or is psychotic or confused.

Research has shown that many people who are diagnosed with depression in the primary care setting do not meet the criteria for a diagnosis of major depression when they are later evaluated by a mental health professional who does a "structured interview" or uses a depression rating scale. Perhaps some of these individuals have less severe symptoms or have mild depression. Sometimes, this results in the overtreatment of elderly people with antidepressant medications when they don't need them. Those individuals would benefit instead from supportive talk therapy (psychotherapy) or counseling or changes to their lifestyle with regular follow-ups. However, if the depression is severe or your loved one is at high risk for suicide or is psychotic, then a referral to a mental health professional is indicated.

You, as a family member, will need to encourage your loved one to comply with the recommended treatment and help to facilitate it by seeing that he fills and takes the prescriptions, assisting with transportation to his appointments, and so forth. If you have any questions about the diagnosis in your senior family member, your family doctor is the best resource to evaluate him and explore further treatment.

TREATMENT

Depression, when accurately diagnosed, should be treated in all persons no matter the age. Sometimes there can be obstacles to receiving treatment in older persons because the senior generation may regard depression as a weakness and are thus reluctant to seek professional help. It's not something they've been accustomed to talking about with others or regarding as an illness.

Older adults who have depression should be encouraged to be physically active and to increase their activity if possible. It's also essential to help your loved one improve her dietary habits and nutrition, increase social interactions by keeping contact with friends, families and social activities, and do the things that bring (or used to bring) her pleasure.

Once the need for treatment is accepted, SSRIs (selective serotonin-reuptake inhibitors) are considered the first-line drug of choice because of their favorable response, low adverse reactions, and low cost. Other medications have also been used successfully (see appendix A). The choice of drug treatment may be difficult because older people are more likely to experience side effects of antidepressant medications. In addition, these drugs may not interact well with her other medications. Age can also lower the body's ability to metabolize antidepressant medications, leading to more side effects. For this reason, many older people quit or forget to take them due to unpleasant side effects, underlying memory problems, or difficulty keeping track of complicated drug schedules. To avoid this problem, electroconvulsive therapy (ECT), or shock therapy, is often recommended as an effective treatment option in this age group. It is the most effective treatment for severely depressed persons, including those who are suicidal, in those who have not responded to other treatments, or those who have a deteriorating physical condition. ECT is administered in a controlled environment (a hospital) and is well tolerated in older persons. The response to ECT occurs within a few weeks, which is much faster than with antidepressant medications.

Psychotherapy is an effective treatment for depression in the elderly and may also be considered a first-line treatment.

TABLE 14.1. Medications with Potential Adverse Effects

MIGHT CAUSE SUICIDAL SYMPTOMS

Pain medications	Acetaminophen/tramadol, hydromorphone, tramadol
Anti-seizure	Carbamazepine, clonazepam, diazepam, ethosuximide, gabapentin, lamotrigine, lorazepam, phenytoin, pregabalin, topiramate, valproic acid, zonisamide
Antidepressants	Amitriptyline, bupropion, citalopram, clomipramine, desipramine, desvenlafaxine, doxepin, duloxetine, escitalopram, fluoxetine/olanzapine, imipramine, mirtazapine, nefazodone, nortriptyline, paroxetine, phenelzine, selegiline, sertraline, trazodone, venlafaxine
Anxiety and sedatives	Alprazolam, butabarbital, chlordiazepoxide, clonazepam, diazepam, doxepin, eszopiclone, flurazepam, pentobarbital, ramelteon, zaleplon, zolpidem
Gastrointestinal	Metoclopramide
Hormones	Finasteride, leuprolide, levonorgestrel, oxandrolone, progesterone
Respiratory	Montelukast, ribavirin, roflumilast, zafirlukast
Other	Acamprosate, amantadine, armodafinil, aripiprazole, asenapine, atomoxetine, carbidopa/levodopa, ciprofloxacin, dapsone, efavirenz, iloperidone, interferon Beta-1a, interferon beta-1b, isoretinoin, lurasidone, memantine, mefloquine, methylphenidate, modafinil, moxifloxacin, naltrexone, olanzapine, ofloxacin, peginterferon alfa 2-a, quetiapine, raltegravir, risperidone, rivastigmine, sibutramine, tetrabenzine, varenicline

TABLE 14.1. **Medications with Potential Adverse Effects** (*continued*)

MIGHT CAUSE DEPRESSIVE SYMPTOMS (NON-SUICIDAL)

Pain medications	Cyclobenzaprine, fentanyl, acetaminophen/hydrocodone, ibuprofen, indomethacin, morphine, nabumetone, oxycodone
Blood pressure medications	Atenolol, betaxolol, bendroflumethiazide/nadolol, brimonidine, brimonidine/timolol, enalapril, hydrochlorothiazide/metoprolol, hydrocodone, metolazone, metoprolol, nisoldipine, quinapril, telmisartan, timolol, trandolapril
Corticosteroids	Betamethasone, cortisone, dexamethasone, methylprednisolone, prednisolone, prednisone, triamcinolone
Gastrointestinal	Atropine/diphenoxylate, cimetidine, dexlansoprazole, esomeprazole, famotidine, omeprazole, ranitidine
Hormones	Anastrozole, bicalutamide, cabergoline, conjugated estrogens, conjugated estrogens/medroxyprogesterone, desoestrel/ ethinyl estradiol, dienogest/estradiol, esterified estrogens, esterified estradiol/levonorgestrel, ethinyl estradiol/ norethindrone, estropipate, ethinyl estradiol/norgestimate, ethinyl estradiol/norgestrel, etonogestrel, exemestane, goserelin, hydroxyprogesterone, medroxyprogesterone, megestrol, norethindrone, tamoxifen, testosterone
Respiratory	Cetirizine
Other	Abacavir/lamivudine, acebutolol, acitretin, amphetamine/ dextroamphetamine, baclofen, benzphetamone, cinacalcet, clonidine, cyclosporine, dantrolene, dexmethylphenidate, donepezil, dronabinol, emtricitabine, erlotinib, flecainide, fluphenazine, galantamine, haloperidol, maraviroc, methyldopa, metolazone, metronidazole, oxybutynin, phentermine, pimozide, prazosin, propafenone, propranolol, rasagiline, rotigotine

Source: Adapted from D. Qato, K. Ozenberger, and M. Olfson, Prevalence of Prescriptions with Depression as a Potential Adverse Effect Among Adults in the United States, *JAMA*, 2018;319(22):2289–2298, doi:10.1001/jama.2018.6741.

WHAT CAN YOU DO?

Beyond the usual supportive strategies described earlier in this book, your primary concern will be to ensure the safety of your loved one. If she lives alone or with a spouse who is also a senior, you want to determine whether she is able to care for herself, bathe, cook, eat, take medications as prescribed, do laundry, get out of the house, and go where she needs to go—to socialize with friends and family, to doctor appointments, to church, or to the grocery store. Participate in life. Endless hours of empty alone time at home are not healthy for anybody. This is where you want to encourage and facilitate her social interactions.

Can he or she walk safely or is he at risk of falling, particularly if a new medication makes him a bit drowsy or he's unsteady? Does he still drive, or should he still be driving in the short term or long term? This is a highly charged question for most families that requires a serious sit-down conversation, with input from his PCP after a thorough neurological exam. Your senior family member should not be driving if he is considered at risk of danger or harm to himself or others. Check your own state's set of definitions and requirements. This is a major decision and affects your loved one's sense of himself as an independent person and his ability to freely engage socially. It takes more effort when he has to take public transportation or depend on rides. Your PCP can assist you with this decision.

If he is unable to do any of these things, can he live alone if you arrange for someone to assist with meals, laundry, and other household tasks? The best way to determine this is to have his PCP evaluate him and have a visiting nurse do a home visit to analyze his living situation and offer a recommendation on what may be needed. He may need a home health aide several hours per week, a move to assisted living, or move in with you or other family members. Remember, though, if everyone is off at work during the day, he may still need an aide during the day or go to an elder day care program so as not to be left home alone. This is particularly important if you think he may be suicidal, when you may also need to have a "sitter" watching and being with him 24/7 until the crisis passes.

Do you think he can reliably take his medications as prescribed, or do you think he becomes confused or is suicidal? These are major questions to address and to revisit often. If you think he becomes confused, does not remember to take his medications, or is so despondent that you cannot trust him and you fear he is suicidal, then he will need continuous observation until this episode passes. You are not alone in making these decisions. They should be done jointly with other family members and his provider and treatment team.

15

What Recovery Looks Like

To understand recovery in your loved one, it's often helpful to look at the impact mood disorders can have on his life. One of the great tragedies of major depression or bipolar disorder is that it often means a *life interrupted*. These chronic and progressive conditions, beginning early in life, may not respond adequately to treatment and often interfere with your loved one's ability to participate fully in life. They can delay educational pursuits, work, and career paths, which then may have to be adjusted because of intolerable stress levels and a decline in cognition (thinking abilities). They can delay personal relationships and many of the natural transitions into adulthood that are put on hold. Underemployment is common, since mood disorders can get in the way of academic and professional advancement; this interference in turn can (temporarily) hinder your loved one's ability to excel in school or work and affect his financial strength. When a mood disorder is linked with other physical medical problems, choices and trade-offs have to be made to manage less than optimal whole-health outcomes.

Impact of Mood Disorders on Life

Impact on natural progression of life events, especially around transition to adulthood

Ability to work, live independently, care for self, manage finances, make decisions

Delay in education, academic performance, achievement or completion

Choice of profession, employer, or job/position (with possible need to take less demanding job or find one that has certain employee benefit programs)

Delayed job or professional advancement

Financial strain

Impaired family, spousal and romantic relationships and friendships

Family responsibilities

Source: Adapted from Depression and Bipolar Support Alliance, *Well Beyond Blue: Report of the Externally Led Patient-Focused Medical Product Development Meeting on Major Depressive Disorder* (DBSA, March 2019).

The Depression and Bipolar Support Alliance (DBSA) became interested in the impact of mood disorders on life and in November 2018 convened a large group of persons living with mood disorders, caregivers, and officials from the US Food and Drug Administration and medical product developers as active listeners. Their goal was to communicate firsthand thoughts, opinions, and perspectives on wellness from patients directly to the decision makers who design and direct research on the drugs and medical products to treat depression. It was part of a 10-year initiative to ensure that affected patient (peer)-derived treatment outcomes be incorporated in the delivery of mental health care for those who have mood disorders, thus giving us a voice in the development of new treatment options. DBSA released a report in March 2019 summarizing the meeting and the results of an online Supporting Wellness survey.

One theme that surfaced in the report was a sense of patient frustration and a belief that "better is not well." There was a strong desire expressed by affected persons to experience a life of being more productive, more financially secure, more engaged in personal relationships and an opportunity to thrive rather than merely function or survive.

RECOVERY

If the goal is to recover from an episode of a mood disorder, to feel better, then you might rightly ask, What will that look like? What is my loved one aiming for? What can we reasonably and realistically expect? Will he or she be able to return to his old life, to school or work, or will he want to? Will he need to take another direction in life? Will she be able to take care of herself, support herself, get a job, have and care for children if she so desires? How involved will I, as the family member, need to be? What if my loved one is doing well and then has a setback? While the specifics are different for each person, there are some common threads in recovery.

WHAT DOES RECOVERY LOOK LIKE?

In recovery, your loved one will have a restored sense of hope and energy. He or she will believe that a return to her life or a satisfying version of her life, away from the symptoms of depression, is possible to achieve, and she will be motivated by that. She will have identified one or more realistic life goals and her unique path to achieve them and is making informed decisions to get there, building on her strengths. She is working toward regaining control over her life. As she recovers, your loved one will develop a new or modified meaning and purpose in life and will strive to reach her full potential regardless of any residual mental health symptoms. Her recovery will involve all aspects of her life—mind, body, spirit, community—and be supported by peers, family, friends, and others who believe in her. This will include positive relationships, with enhanced community and ways to spend her time in work, family, social, or volunteer roles. Respect, with decreased stigma and discrimination, will be assumed. Well-being will be an overall goal.

Recovery from an episode of mental illness looks a little different for each person. It has been defined in several ways. It's not the 12-Step Recovery program (created by the founders of Alcoholics Anonymous) that you might have heard of, which is wonderful and designed for the specific purpose of recovery from alcohol and substance use disorders. The objective in recovery from a mental illness like a mood disorder is to be able to function in life as each one of us defines it. It's a lifelong process in which the person strives to participate fully in life, even in the presence of continuing residual (leftover) symptoms. Recovery is often thought of as reducing (or eliminating) depression symptoms with a return to function. People who have depression or bipolar disorder should be able to live their lives in a way that is symptom-free and allows them to participate in their chosen (healthy) life activities and relationships.

NAMI (National Alliance of Mental Illness) reminds us that recovery is a process, beginning with diagnosis and eventually moving into the successful management of a mental health condition. It's an ongoing process. Sustained recovery involves

- learning about the illness and effective treatment (and engaging in that treatment),
- becoming empowered with the support of peers and family members, and
- for some, helping others achieve wellness.

Most people diagnosed with a mental health condition can experience relief from their symptoms and live a satisfying life by actively participating in an individualized treatment plan. An effective treatment plan may include medication, psychotherapy, and peer support groups. A balanced diet, exercise, and sleep can also play a big role in one's mental health. Meaningful social opportunities and volunteer activities contribute to overall wellness and mental health recovery.

One definition of recovery that I like is: "The ongoing process of regaining control of your life after a psychiatric diagnosis, and all of the losses that accompany it" (DBSA/Appalachian Consulting Group, 2009). I'm drawn to this definition because it emphasizes recovery as an *ongoing process*, not a static event with a limited time frame, a specific beginning and an end. That suits the nature of mood disorders. *Regaining control of your life* seems to resonate with many people I speak with in groups who often feel that their lives are out of their immediate control during an episode of depression or mania, following a direction they do not want. It feels to them as though the illness is controlling their lives, which are filled with depression symptoms, therapy appointments, and struggles to get through the day. So, regaining control is a worthy goal. And we usually do not think of the losses that accompany a psychiatric diagnosis, yet they can have a powerful influence on our lives. What do I mean by losses?

There are many different types of losses that may occur in your loved one's life during a time like this, when his life and world is dramatically changed by experiencing a mental illness. These losses can be different for each person. Some common examples include

- loss of the way he sees or defines himself after receiving a psychiatric diagnosis
- loss of self-esteem
- loss of friendship and personal relationships, including with a spouse or significant other
- loss of pleasure and enjoyment in life
- loss of time from his life
- loss of productivity
- loss of school or work
- loss of a job
- financial losses, due to the loss of income from not working as much, medical bills, or excessive spending sprees during a manic episode
- lost opportunities
- other losses

The effect of these losses added together can have a profound negative impact on a person's life if he or she does not acknowledge them and deal with them directly. How does your loved one do that? First, the person needs to recognize and grieve the losses. He needs to take some time to ponder the loss and its impact on him, sit with it for a while, mull it over a bit without obsessing about it, allow himself to feel the sadness and sorrow of the loss for a while. Then he must put it aside and not think about it constantly. This is the healthy response to loss. If he does not do this, it will pop up to haunt him at the most unlikely moments.

Another working definition of recovery that is often cited, offered by the Substance Abuse and Mental Health Services Administration (SAMHSA), was created jointly by a group of professionals and stakeholders in August 2010: "A process of change through which individuals improve their health and wellness, live a self-directed life, and strive to reach their full -potential." The important pieces to this definition are first that it's an *ongoing process of change.* There is no quick fix or magic pill, and unfortunately no specific end point in sight after which she no longer has to pay attention or do any work to stay well. Don't be discouraged by this. Recovery has an overall upward course marked by little ups and downs in each day or week, with occasional plateaus where your family member might feel as though she is not making any progress at all. That makes it more difficult to stick with a treatment plan and recovery goals but improvement will occur, and she'll be glad that she persevered. It's based on continual growth, with occasional setbacks, and learning from experience. Eventually, paying attention to his or her mental health will become habit and will not feel like a lifelong burden.

The next point to this definition is that *you* do it; you're the one to accomplish these things. It's not done *to* you. Your loved one doesn't sit by passively in therapy or as a patient and take some magic pill without doing some degree of recovery work, actively participating in the process.

Recovery involves a change in something he does or the way he does it that will result in improving his health and wellness, live a life as he wants it to be, and reach his full potential. Change is based on dissatisfaction in some area of his life that motivates him to take action. Maybe it's a change in the way he thinks about himself and the world; a change in the negative thoughts he has; a change away from toxic people, situations, or habits that drag him down; a change in his diet and exercise habits—maybe he stops smoking or drinking alcohol. Change can sometimes feel odd at first, as it may involve moving out of his comfort zone to reach his goals. The best advice is to start in small steps and keep his goals in mind. The SAMHSA definition of recovery is guided by four major features that support a life in recovery:

Health: managing general physical health and well-being; this involves managing all of one's physical and mental illnesses, or symptoms, including alcohol and substance use and addiction. It includes making informed, healthy choices that support physical and emotional well-being that will sustain ongoing recovery.

Home: having a stable and safe place to live, one that is consistent and peaceful that will help remove uncertainty and anxiety in life that can lead to self-destructive behavior.

Purpose: having meaningful daily activities and being productive, such as in a job, school, volunteer position, family caretaking, or creative endeavors and having the independence, income, and resources to participate in society.

Community: having relationships and social networks that provide non-judgmental support, friendship, love, and hope.

To enhance the definition, SAMHSA has offered 10 guiding principles of mental health recovery:

Recovery emerges from hope. The belief that recovery is real and possible provides the essential and motivating message of a better future that people can overcome the internal and external challenges, barriers, and obstacles and move on. Hope is the catalyst of the recovery process upon which all else is built. Peers, families, friends, providers, and others can help foster hope.

Recovery involves self-direction. People define their own life goals and design their unique life paths toward those goals. In this way, self-determination and self-direction are the foundations of recovery. Individuals optimize their autonomy (ability to make independent decisions and not be controlled in what they do, think, and feel) and independence by leading, controlling, and exercising choice over the mental health services and supports that assist their recovery. This is empowering. They are provided the resources to make informed decisions, initiate recovery, build on their strengths, and gain or regain control over their lives. They determine their own path of recovery with their autonomy, independence, and control of resources.

Recovery occurs via many individualized pathways. There are multiple pathways to recovery based on an individual's unique strengths as well as his or her unique needs, preferences, goals, culture, background, and experiences, including trauma experience. Recovery is built on the many capacities, strengths, talents, coping abilities, resources, and inherent value of each person. Recovery pathways are highly personalized and may include professional treatment, medications, family support, school support, faith-based approaches, peer-support, and others. Recovery is not a step-by step formula but one based on continual growth, with occasional setbacks and learning from experience.

Recovery is holistic. Recovery encompasses an individual's whole life, including mind, body, spirit, and community. Recovery embraces all aspects of life, including self-care practices, mental health and primary health care treatment, dental care, faith, spirituality, creativity, family supports and social networks, housing, employment, education, and transportation.

Recovery is supported by peers and allies. Mutual support plays an invaluable role in recovery. Individuals encourage and engage others in recovery and provide one another with a sense of belonging, supportive relationships, and community.

Recovery is supported through relationships and social networks. The presence and involvement of people who believe in the person's ability to recover; offer hope, support, and encouragement; and suggest strategies and resources for change. These are important in the recovery process. This includes family members, peers, providers, faith groups, community members, and others. Through these relationships, people leave unhealthy roles behind and engage in new life roles that lead to a greater sense of belonging, person, empowerment, autonomy, social inclusion, and community participation.

Recovery is culturally based. Culture and cultural background (values, traditions, beliefs) are key in determining a person's pathway to recovery. Mental health care services should be culturally grounded, attuned, sensitive, congruent, and personalized to meet each individual's unique needs.

Recovery is supported by addressing trauma. The experience of trauma (physical or emotional) is often a precursor to or associated with alcohol or drug use, mental health problems, and relational issues. Services and supports should be trauma-informed for safety and trust as well as to promote choice, empowerment, and collaboration.

Recovery is strengths based. The strengths and resources of individuals, families, and communities serve as the foundation of recovery. Recovery focuses on valuing and building on the multiple capacities, resiliencies, talents, coping abilities, and inherent worth of individuals. The process of recovery moves forward through interaction with others in supportive, trust-based relationships. Each person has a personal responsibility for their own self-care and recovery journey, identifying coping strategies and healing processes to promote their own wellness. Families and significant others have a responsibility to support their loved ones, and communities have a responsibility to provide opportunities and resources to foster social inclusion and recovery.

Recovery is based on respect. Eliminating discrimination and stigma are crucial in achieving recovery. This includes acceptance on a community, systems, and society level and ensures that rights are protected. Self-acceptance, developing a positive and meaningful sense of identity, and regaining belief in oneself are particularly vital.

Source: SAMHSA. *SAMHSA's Working Definition of Recovery: 10 Guiding Principles of Recovery.* 2012. https://store.samhsa.gov/system/files/pep12-recdef.pdf

Another definition of "personal" recovery follows: "Recovery is described as a deeply personal, unique process of changing one's attitudes, values, feelings, goals, skills, and/or roles. It is a way of living a satisfying, hopeful, and contributing life even within the limitations caused by illness. Recovery involves the development of new meaning and purpose in one's life as one grows beyond the catastrophic effects of mental illness" (Anthony 1993, 4). This definition is interesting because it emphasizes that one can have a satisfying life despite experiencing the symptoms of mental illness or a mood disorder. He or she can grow beyond the episode and its effects. It's an important point to remember. Your family member can *thrive* despite and beyond their diagnosis. Sometimes it's in a new dimension or capacity, but it's not as grim as things may appear today.

THE RECOVERY PROCESS

Recovery is a long-term, ongoing process, with many ups and downs and occasional setbacks from which one learns. Recovery does not happen in a nice straight line from illness to wellness with a clear endpoint. Instead, it looks more like a zigzag pattern with forward progress and occasional setbacks. It occurs in small steps. Then, suddenly, there are some plateaus or times when it appears as though nothing is happening. This is very frustrating for everyone, and it's a time when your support for your loved one is particularly important.

> Recovery is a long-term, ongoing process. But it *is* possible.

If your loved one has a depression that has been difficult to treat, or he is in a treatment-resistant category, he may feel that recovery is very far away and does not even apply to him. It gets quite discouraging, and many people reach the point where they want to give up trying. Yet, just because recovery is difficult does not mean that it's impossible. It's just more of a challenge, and more of a reward when progress is eventually made. Your job is to be creative in your support efforts and to offer *realistic optimism*, which is a reasonable view of the future that involves hope and the confidence that things will turn out well, with enough hard work and determination. This is hard to hold on to.

Recovery needs to be managed, and it takes time to learn how to do that. Sorry, but there is no quick fix for recovery from a mental illness. This makes it sound disheartening. Here's where persistence, hard work, and trust in a good treatment team can make a world of difference.

When you think about recovery, you have to think about the obstacles all around us in life that are there to trip us up. We have to find ways to work around them. These obstacles can come from internal or external sources. An *internal obstacle* could be a negative thought your family member has ("I'm always bad at _____") or a way of thinking that gets in the way of her recovery. External events at work or in social situations, or other people's thoughts and comments, may also present obstacles and impact her decisions. Perhaps your loved one might have heard: "Why are you seeing that therapist? You don't need to go!" That is an obstacle to his or her recovery.

Being aware of something that is an obstacle is the first step in controlling them, as it allows her to change her course and take steps to avoid or decrease the influence that the situation or person may have on her. In this way, it diminishes the negative impact on your loved one's recovery path that the obstacle *could* have had.

Another thing to consider is, How will he or she know when he is moving forward in recovery? You don't want to wait six months for an "ah-ha" moment—that's too long to wait for a moment to be motivating and it could get discouraging in between.

Offer realistic optimism.

The answer is have him look for the little markers along the way, small indications that he is getting back to his usual self. Perhaps he notices that he's starting to return phone calls more often, or he picks up the phone and initiates a call to a friend or makes plans for lunch or hanging out. Or she's resumed interest in a previous hobby or pastime that was put aside because of her depression. Perhaps others have mentioned that she's been smiling or laughing a bit on occasion. Your loved one needs to pay attention to these little things and not disregard them as insignificant—they are important markers in the path to recovery. She might make a point of noting the times when these things happen and use them to inspire, encourage, and motivate her to keep going on the days that seem glum.

Look for the small indications of the return of your loved one's usual self.

An example of a person in recovery from depression is seen in the following story about Luke.

> Luke is a 31-year-old man who has been receiving treatment for major depressive disorder for the past several years. He is a technical high school graduate and works in the town utility company. Luke went through many different types of treatments, including antidepressant medications and talk therapy and has had one inpatient hospitalization. He regularly attends Alcoholics Anonymous meetings, as he initially tried to self-medicate his depression with excess alcohol and is now proud of his five-year sobriety. At its worst, Luke felt that all he was doing was spending time thinking about how to manage his depression and trying to hide it from his co-workers and friends. He took a leave of absence from work, during which time he received regular mental health treatment. But it seemed that dealing with this illness and going to these many appointments were taking up all of his time. He was also worn out by trying to fend off his family who kept asking how he was doing. He lost touch with his friends and interest in biking and other things he used to like.
>
> Luke is now doing better, thanks to his ability to stick to his treatment plan and trust in his providers. The negative thoughts, which had once ruled his life, are now gone, replaced by more realistic and optimistic ones.

He has more confidence in himself and what he can do, with a sense of purpose and direction in his days and can now stand up to the criticisms of his controlling father. Luke now has hope for his future, both personally and at work, and is making plans to get another state certification in his field. He has hope that this might lead to a better position and possible promotion at work; he is making the best use of his technical skills and believes he deserves it. Luke has started exercising again on his bike, is eating more healthy food choices and has dropped eight pounds without trying. His family has learned about his illness and how to be supportive, and that is a huge relief. Luke has reconnected with two of his old friends, and also has plans to propose to his girlfriend, something he had not thought possible when depressed. All in all, he is now functioning in his life again in a way that he defines and is managing the ups and downs of life with greater ease.

WELL-BEING

Well-being is the ultimate goal in recovery from a mood disorder. It is possible and realistic for those of us who have depression to expect well-being—this I know for sure. What is well-being? The concept and definitions of wellness and illness have changed from the mid-twentieth century until now. The definition of mental illness has changed from focusing on the *diagnosis* of mental illness to focusing on the *person*. It has also transitioned from an *absence of disease* model to one that stresses positive psychological function for mental health.

This means that the absence of symptoms is not enough to feel well. Being well is not only freedom from the episodes of a mood disorder or depression symptoms. It's an ongoing process that includes participating in the world around you, being in control of your life, and having a sense of personal growth and relationships that matter. It means that your loved one has a sense of competence and mastery in the things he does in his life and that he feels good about who he is.

The psychologist C. D. Ryff, from the University of Wisconsin–Madison, defines wellness and well-being and reminds us that the absence of mental distress does not guarantee we will experience well-being. This is a very important point. In addition, we need to be mindful that mental health is intertwined with physical health, and positive mental health may influence good physical health and biological functioning. This means that the health of our bodies and brains are linked together. A type of psychotherapy called *well-being therapy*, which has a focus on positive experience and learning how to savor those positive experiences, has been linked with improved symptoms of depression.

There is an interesting article on psychological well-being by Ryff (2014) called "Psychological Well-Being Revisited: Advances in Science and Practice" (2014). In the past, psychologists thought of well-being as happiness, satisfaction with life, and a positive affect (which is similar to mood). Thinking about it in another way, Ryff describes the essential features of well-being as follows:

- *Having a purpose in life*, feeling your life has meaning and direction. You might find this in your work or volunteer activities, as a student, parent, or in whatever role guides you. Our purpose is easy to forget when we're depressed, so we do have to work at it.
- *Living a life based on your own personal convictions*, beliefs, opinions, and principles. This means you are free to make decisions for yourself (called *autonomy*). For example, if you are an adult, do you feel controlled by another person, or respected for your thoughts, opinions, and decisions?
- *Making use of your personal talents and potential*, also called *personal growth*. This growth could occur in your work, school, volunteering, or family life.
- *Managing your life situations well*, also called mastering your environment. We all experience fluctuations, the ups and downs of daily life: the key is how we learn to deal with them.
- *Having positive relationships* with deep ties to others. Your close personal connections could be with friends or family members—just as long as you have them. These relationships are important to maintaining your mental health balance and definitely help with depression, a time when isolation can occur.
- *Accepting yourself*, which means having knowledge and accepting who you are as a person, including your own limitations. Nobody's perfect. We all have our own strengths and weaknesses, and we do better when we learn to accept and work with them.

In conclusion, your loved one in recovery will have a life that is meaningful to her, with purpose and direction, that is based on her own beliefs and convictions, making use of her personal talents and potential, where she will manage her life situations well, have positive relationships, and accept herself. This is what recovery will look like.

16

Anticipating Recovery: Skills to Have in Place

RESILIENCE

Perhaps you have heard the saying, "Build your life raft before you need it." You might wonder what that has to do with mood disorders, particularly with your family member or friend who has depression. *Life raft* refers to the coping and adaptive skills people have successfully used to manage life and depression. Here, it means you encourage your family member or friend to learn these coping skills now, when he feels well, so they are available to him in the future when depression symptoms strike.

> **Resilience indicates the ability to bounce back more readily after adversity.**

Why is this important? Those who cope effectively with the negative effects of stress and their illness may "bounce back" more readily after an episode of depression or bipolar disorder. This is known as *resilience*, defined in the online brochure *The Road to Resilience* by the American Psychological Association (APA) (www.apa.org/helpcenter/road-resilience.aspx) as the "process of adapting well in the face of adversity, trauma, threats, and significant sources of stress—such as family and relationship problems, serious health problems, or workplace and financial stress."

Think of resilience as an ongoing way of dealing with the difficult times in our lives, facing challenges (such as an illness like depression or bipolar disorder), finding solutions, and recovering from setbacks. Having resilience means that your loved one learns effective ways of thinking and responding during difficult situations. Resilience involves having adaptive behaviors and coping skills, such as problem solving, managing stress, facing one's fears, mastering challenges, regulating one's emotions, and learning the consequences of one's behaviors. These coping strategies can help a person survive and thrive despite hardship.

Resilience includes hope for recovery and a sense of determination. Adapting to stress and difficult life events is a complicated process. We learn some of it from our parents and family. It is also likely that genetic factors influence our resilience to adversity. On the other hand, resilience doesn't require a person to have exceptional or unique traits. Rather, it comes from the common inner qualities that surface when we adapt to stress.

You might wonder what makes some people more resilient than others. Southwick and Charney (2012) looked at this very question. They surveyed three groups of people who had experienced extraordinary adversity in life and who survived remarkably well. In the survey responses, they found ten personal characteristics or coping strategies common to those in each of these three groups. They found that people who have resilience used many of these strategies, which they call *Resilience Factors*. They are presented for you here in table 16.1.

In addition, *The Road to Resilience* brochure (APA 2013) from the APA identifies the following coping strategies. They are considered important in your loved one's efforts to develop resilience, meaning that those who have these traits seem to have an easier time bouncing back from adversity:

- Avoid seeing crises as insurmountable. Develop confidence in your ability to solve problems.
- Accept change as a part of living.
- Make connections.
- Make realistic goals and move toward them.
- Take decisive action in difficult situations.
- Look for opportunities for self-discovery.
- Nurture a positive view of yourself. Trust your own instincts.
- Keep things in perspective.
- Maintain a hopeful outlook.
- Take care of yourself. Maintain flexibility and balance in life.

The APA also notes that caring and supportive relationships, inside and outside the family, are essential to building resilience. They create love and trust, provide role models, and offer encouragement. You'll also see there are resilience characteristics common to the two lists I just presented to you.

People tend to use various approaches to learn resilience skills. The choice depends on the individual person, the resources he has available through family and friends, and the characteristics of his culture, religion, and community. The culture or community a person was raised in might influence whether and how much he connects with others, communicates his feelings, or deals with adversity. Some people are very private and uncomfortable sharing their feelings, while others reveal every last detail of their emotional life.

TABLE 16.1. **Resilience Factors**
1. Maintain an optimistic but realistic outlook.
2. Confront your fears.
3. Rely on your inner core values and altruism.
4. Draw on religious or spiritual practices.
5. Seek and accept social support.
6. Imitate resilient role models.
7. Attend to your physical, mental, and emotional health and well-being.
8. Challenge your mind to maintain brain fitness.
9. Try to maintain cognitive and emotional flexibility—accept that which you cannot change and focus on what you can change.
10. Look for meaning, purpose, and opportunity in the face of adversity.

Source: S. M. Southwick and D. S. Charney, *Resilience: The Science of Mastering Life's Greatest Challenges* (Cambridge University Press, 2012).

What does all of this mean, and how does it apply to your family member or friend? It means that, in trying to support and encourage resilience in your loved one (her ability to bounce back after adversity like an episode of mental illness), you use a variety of methods. Customize them to your skills and what you think your loved one will respond to. You might choose one or a few of the tactics outlined in table 16.1, such as "being a positive role model" yourself or "maintaining an optimistic but realistic look" at her situation, combined with one or two items in the *Road to Resilience* list on the preceding page like "keeping things in perspective." Then add in your own life experiences to create a plan to help develop resilience in your loved one. You might focus on helping her develop confidence in her ability to take decisive action and solve problems.

The following story of Angie shows us how a person can experience adversity, such as an episode of bipolar depression, and have the skills and personal qualities to bounce back.

Angie is a 37-year-old woman who has a long history of bipolar disorder, having had numerous episodes of the ups and downs that come along with this illness. At first, she was devastated after an episode of her illness had come and gone and felt as if her life was meaningless and without hope or purpose. She found that it took months for her to get back on her feet, with many leftover or residual symptoms of depression haunting her. Angie had a hard time keeping a job, since stigma made her too embarrassed to approach her supervisor and explain her illness, and she was let go for too many unexplained absences.

Over time, Angie learned how best to manage her bipolar depression and hypomania, and she worked with her therapist and family on ways to improve her ability to bounce back—her resilience. She learned to stay in touch with her healthy baseline self, with who she is as a person, and not forget that she has personal skills and value, understanding that her illness does not define her. Angie also learned how to contain her impulses and to problem solve difficult situations. She tried to keep a reasonable, realistic view of her future and eventually learned that, with enough hard work, support, and treatment, things would improve. She did not have this confidence before; it felt good and gave her a sense of hope. Angie was able to focus on a few concrete and realistic goals for her future and took some computer skills classes in anticipation of applying for a new job, building on her strengths and personal qualities. Her family encouraged her and were optimistic that she would succeed. It also required having a more positive view of herself.

Angie reached out to her close friends and family for support and convinced them to learn about her illness; they then were able to offer the support and encouragement she needed. They also kept her mindful of her inner strengths that got her through previous episodes in the past. In addition, she paid greater attention to caring for her personal self and her mind, eating a healthy diet, getting enough sleep, participating in daily physical exercise, and solving puzzles, Sudoku, and other games to keep her mind sharp.

Once she had mastered these things, Angie found that six months later when she had another episode of depression (sadly, recurrence is characteristic of her illness) it appeared to be shorter and less intense. She was also able to return to her baseline functioning self more quickly after the episode and had fewer residual (leftover) symptoms to bother her. It was easier for her to bounce back.

Using the Resilience Factors described on the preceding pages, here are some ways you can help your loved one build resilience. The hope is that these skills will lend him a greater ability to face the challenges of his illness and recover more readily when mood fluctuations occur. He may also be better able to manage stress and feelings of anxiety.

HOW TO HELP YOUR LOVED ONE
BUILD RESILIENCE

There are many strategies that can help your loved one build resilience. Many of them are listed next. Don't think that you have to master all of them. Instead, choose one or two you feel may work for your family member and give them a try. If they don't work or they are too hard to do, choose another one or two.

- Provide unconditional, *nonjudgmental love and support*. It's important to support your family member or friend as he works to build resilience.
- Maintain an *optimistic but realistic outlook* for your family member or friend with depression. This means holding a reasonable view of the future that involves hope and the confidence that things will turn out well, with enough hard work. Then help your family member or friend embrace this realistic attitude about his future. Help him avoid having unattainable dreams as goals. Focus on what he can do now with effort and encouragement. It may be difficult, but try to remain hopeful about his future. No one can predict the course of anyone's depression or recovery. I've often been reminded that you can never know what's around the corner, what will happen next, whether it's a new treatment for mood disorders or a positive life event. Encourage him to continue with his chosen path in life, even if at a slower pace for now. Sometimes, one's life plans have to be put on hold for a little while during an illness. Consider it a temporary pause and not the final stop.
- Keep an *optimistic attitude* when your family member's or friend's moods fluctuate. You may find this very hard to do. Try the following:
  - Remind him that this situation won't last forever.
  - Help him *keep the illness or negative event in perspective*. Remind him that, although depression is a biological illness that's a part of his life, it does not *define* him.
  - *Confront his negative thoughts and emotions* using the method from chapter 8. Encourage him to recall past achievements to find evidence for the positive and evidence against his negative views of himself and the world. Urge him to seek an outside opinion of himself from those he respects. Positive thinking (including hopefulness and a positive view of himself and the world) and positive life events can act as a buffer against depression symptoms in vulnerable people.

- Have your family member or friend *recall the inner strengths and resources* he has used to deal with problems in the past. Encourage him to use them now. His perseverance or sense of humor might help him through a difficult time.
  - *Bring up past successes* that obviously show his strengths and abilities. Then offer him new opportunities to demonstrate those strengths and reinforce his confidence.
- Guide your family member or friend toward *concrete and realistic goals.* Urge him to plan his future in small, incremental steps. Encourage him to gain the skills to reach his goal, gather the support he needs, and take the action to succeed.
- Be supportive as your family member or friend learns to *face his fears.* Fear can interfere with moving forward and recovering from depression. It may be helpful if he first accepts his fears, gathers information about them, and then makes plans to confront them. Many people find this far better than passively wishing them away.
- Help him *guide his life by the core values* he has learned over time and the benefits he has received from reaching out to help others. *Core values* are the principles, such as honesty, respect, fairness, and compassion, by which we lead our lives. Remind him to rely on his inner sense of right and wrong (his *moral compass*) during periods of stress. Suggest he practice altruism, the act of helping others. Volunteering can bring great benefits as he works to build resilience.
- Consider whether a *spiritual or religious approach* is useful for your loved one. Southwick and Charney (2012) found that some people turn to religion or spirituality to cope with adversity. This approach, they discovered, can lead to lower levels of depression and restore hope and a more balanced view.
- Increase your family member's or friend's *social support network.* This is a foundation on which to build resilience. Close relationships build strength and may protect him during stressful times. Isolation and decreased social support frequently lead to increased stress and depression.
- *Become a role model* for your loved one as a tool to increase his resilience. Family members and caregivers often play the role model who demonstrates skills and behaviors your family member or friend may imitate. Role models help build resilience through their words and actions. Role models can help guide a person as he learns to manage stress; handle disappointment, difficult life situations, and relationships; make major decisions; and care for himself physically and

emotionally. You might try the following techniques (Southwick and Charney 2012):

- Provide consistent and reliable support.
- Inspire and motivate him by your actions.
- Foster self-esteem.
- Model right versus wrong.
- Show how to handle difficult situations.
- Model (show) how to control impulses.
- Advise how to delay gratification and soothe oneself.
- Demonstrate how to take responsibility for oneself and one's own actions.

- Encourage your family member or friend to take care of his *physical and cognitive self* (his mind) and learn self-care. Following a daily physical exercise program is important. Regular exercise acts as an aid to depression treatment and lends a sense of self-confidence and self-respect. Physical training helps to improve mood, thinking, self-confidence, and emotional resilience. It also improves mental and emotional health and well-being and decreases the symptoms of depression. In addition to physical exercise, daily brain activity keeps the mind sharp and ready to face life's challenges. Encourage your family member or friend to read, solve puzzles or games like Sudoku, or play challenging mind games rather than sit aimlessly on the couch in front of the television.

> **Help your loved one find a purpose in life.**

- Help your family member or friend *accept* what he cannot change and focus on what he can do now. Remind him that change is a part of living. Certain goals may no longer be attainable as a result of his illness.

- Support your family member or friend as he *learns to control and tolerate* his strong feelings, emotions, and impulses. This is frequently done with a therapist, but a family member can reinforce it at home.

- Encourage your family member or friend to *seek a purpose* in life rather than aimlessly wandering from one school or job to the next. How do you do this? Help him find something he enjoys and does well. Support him in completing a required educational or training program. This could involve school, work, family, sports, social service, or volunteer activities.

- Help him identify and *build on the strengths and personal qualities* he already has. Sometimes depression makes it difficult for a person to see these qualities in himself. Try using the strategies outlined in chapter 8.

- Work with your family member or friend as he develops new *problem-solving skills*. Reinforce those he already has. See chapter 9 for an outline of ideas to encourage problem solving.

If your family member or friend is temporarily unable to think clearly or experiences depression, hopelessness, and lack of energy, he may find it hard to learn the new skills needed to build resilience. Although his overwhelming thinking is often negative, his self-confidence may diminish, and his ability to manage strong feelings frequently wanes, these skills aren't impossible to learn. It often just takes the right timing and perseverance on his part.

17

Caring for the Caregivers

YOU

After attempting many of the things mentioned in this book to help your family member or friend who has depression or bipolar disorder, you may feel emotionally and physically exhausted. You may also find that her illness personally affects you in other ways. Perhaps you fear that you may have done something to cause your family member's unhappiness. Perhaps you fear you said something that set her into a tailspin. In addition, the interactions you have with her may be difficult and stressful. This could be for several reasons.

Those who experience depression often have trouble reciprocating in a relationship. If that's the case, you may find it challenging to keep giving of yourself when you are receiving little in return. You may offer love but feel it's not returned, you may offer compassion but be told "you don't understand," or you may offer support but be told it's not enough or not the "right kind." This can make you feel guilty, then angry, and then guilty for feeling angry.

Caregivers sometimes become frustrated with their family member or friend for her behavior and mood swings. You may feel ready to abruptly say, "Snap out of it!" You may wonder why your mother or spouse or son puts you through an emotional roller coaster by being inconsistently irritable or stopping his medications. This can lead to anger and may destroy relationships.

You may eventually start feeling bad about yourself. You may feel sad, begin to doubt your abilities, or feel helpless at your inability to solve your family member's problems. Some caregivers develop depression themselves, related to the caregiving or independent of that activity. (If you are concerned that you have depression, see the last part of this chapter.) You may come to resent your friend or family member and then grow angry toward her. Or maybe you desire to escape the situation entirely. This can make you think you are selfish and unloving, which is certainly not true. If you find yourself in a difficult situation with your loved one, you may need to take a break from the moment. Go outside for a walk or do something to care for yourself. A weekend or a week away is great, but you can't always do that.

Illness in a family member may influence you and your family's day-to-day routine, social activities, opportunities, finances, and personal relationships. Taking care of someone who has depression can be a full-time job. Everything seems to stop to accommodate her emotional issues and scheduled appointments. This can be emotionally and physically exhausting on you and on other family members, and you feel drained.

Perhaps the time you spend enjoying your own friends and other relatives has been put on hold because your family member's illness takes priority. You may even lose friends if they are unable to understand depression as a biologically based illness and the responsibilities you have with your loved one. You may also feel guilty engaging in your own hobbies, other interests, or self-care activities and thus stop doing them.

> Caretaking is a full-time job.

I urge you to not let the presence of illness in the family interfere with your social connectedness. Do your best to keep up with your own friends, other family members, hobbies, activities, and social events *without* feeling guilty. Make your own self-care a priority. You need these things in your life to sustain you and maintain your own healthy mental state. This will also allow you to be a better caretaker in the long run.

Changes in Your Life as a Caretaker

A lot will change in your life when you assume the role of caretaker for your family member who has a mood disorder. He or she will probably be in the front of your mind, with concerns about her well-being and safety, treatments, medications, daily activities, and other life decisions. There will likely be changes in your

- family life and routine
- peace and peace of mind
- personal space
- finances (increased medical bills, groceries, transportation, nonmedical expenses)
- sleep
- time: for your own self-care, physical exercise, activities, hobbies
- leisure, relaxation, ability to sit and relax, think, read
- personal relationships, visitors, friendships, which may dwindle
- things that make life meaningful for you and decrease your stress

You will need to be aware of these changes and take steps to see that your usual daily routines and those of the family are maintained and protected and that there are emotional outlets and supports in place for yourself and your other family members. This will take a period of adjustment and can be unsettling. It takes time to get used to the changes associated with the extra effort of caregiving. You will have to plan ways for your family to relax and get away from the caregiver role at times. And remember to treat your loved one who has a mood disorder normally and, as much as possible, include her in normal daily activities and family outings.

You will need to plan for a change in your financial resources that may be consumed in caring for her medical care or daily needs. Financially supporting someone else has an impact on your personal expenses, and you may need a new budget. You may also need to consider whether you can claim these expenses on your income taxes with him or her as a dependent. This is a question for an accountant or a financial advisor.

If your loved one now lives in the same household as you, you will need to consider the impact on the rest of the family. How do they feel about someone coming back to live with you (an adult child or a parent)? A new person in the house adds burdens and stress even in the best situations. If it's a senior parent coming to live with you, how will your children's or teenagers' activities affect your parent? And how will your parent's presence affect them? How does your spouse feel about this? This may be particularly tense if your marriage is already under stress. All people who are affected need to be involved in the decision and have the opportunity to express their feelings and concerns initially and as things go along.

Pace Yourself

I heard a very good piece of advice from a dear friend of mine who is dealing with his 20-something daughter's severe depression. While at first he hoped to see her recover in two to three months, that was not to be. He and his wife learned that life was a marathon, not a sprint, and that ultimate patience was required on their part. They have learned that it's essential to *pace yourself* when you have a loved one who's struggling with this illness. Pacing yourself means doing only what you can realistically do, in reasonable steps and small bites with periodic breathers. Try not to do or be everything for everybody. Their sage advice offers you protection from burnout and from responding to your loved one in a way that you might later regret.

Depression affects the entire family in many ways, and one's efforts to help without being controlling or taking over her life requires a lot of energy.

There is constant worry and concern, and a sense of feeling powerless to make things better, each of which can be all consuming and sometimes overwhelming. As a parent, family member, or close friend, you might feel a need to take on total responsibility and be there as a constant companion, see that she eats, do the laundry, schedule appointments, and provide transportation. You might be tempted to excuse her of responsibilities or shared chores at home, absolve her of obligations, including those at school or work, and perhaps support him or her financially in the long term. But wait—this is not the best approach.

> You need to pace yourself as you struggle to help your loved one.

I'm not suggesting that you put your loved one out on the street in a crisis. I am asking you to think about what is in the best interest of your family member and what is realistic for you to offer. While some of these ideas may be helpful in the short term, overall many of them are not healthy for your loved one in the long run; it won't help him get back on his feet and care for himself after an episode or series of episodes. There's a fine line that you must be aware of between supporting your family member and making him totally dependent on you. You want to provide for him yet allow him to be as self-sufficient as is realistic. A therapist or your family doctor may be helpful in making these difficult decisions.

So, you have to pace yourself and allow your family member to learn how to live with his illness, make mistakes, and thrive. This is very hard to do. Learn your own realistic limitations without feeling guilty. Be supportive. Make sure he has the essentials to live and that he receives professional mental and physical health treatment. Do *some* things but resist the urge to do everything for him. And take care of yourself properly, with the same kindness you would extend to others. Caring for yourself and pacing yourself will help you avoid burnout, which is discussed later in this chapter.

THE FAMILY

The vulnerability of a depressed person and the stability of the family are often connected. If the family has serious issues or family members have medical or mental illnesses themselves, depression in their loved one is likely to worsen or take longer to resolve. Families often vary in their ability to adapt to stress. Some families cope well; some, not so well. Their social and financial resources, the family makeup, the availability of social support, and the presence of other illnesses may influence this. The family's inability to respond adequately to stress may prolong a person's depression episode.

Many families experience a financial strain when one of them suffers from a mental illness. This could be due to loss of income if your ill family member is no longer as productive and has stopped working. Caring for her may have forced you to cut back on your own work hours. Treatment expenses for medications, appointments, and therapy, some of which may not be fully covered by your health insurance, contribute to the financial strain. Add to that transportation costs, taking time off for appointments, or providing day care for your children while you attend these appointments. All of that all builds up.

Depression in a Partner

If your family member who has depression is a spouse or a partner, other factors may affect your relationship. You may start assuming different roles, with the healthy person taking on more responsibility for the household duties, family, and the relationship. Your daily routine and social life may change—fun and laughter might be a fading memory. With more of the daily and financial responsibilities on your shoulders, when you're fatigued you could come to resent being put in that position. You could have intimacy and sexual difficulties as well. This can result from the depression and side effects of some of the medications used to treat it. If your marriage or relationship had troubles before your loved one's illness, they may continue or grow worse now. Take this opportunity to openly communicate with your partner and have her speak with her provider about the problem.

You, as the healthy one, may feel a loss and a sense of isolation since your depressed loved one is not as available to you as in the past. You don't seem to enjoy each other's company as before, and meaningful conversations are a thing of the past. She may not be as emotionally available to you to help solve family, relationship, or child-rearing issues or to make household decisions. This can extend to other social relationships that you once enjoyed together, and you now feel distanced from them, adding to your sense of isolation.

If neither of you recognize that she is experiencing clinical depression, you may wonder why she's behaving so negatively and is withdrawn or irritable. Is she angry with you? A depressed person's fatigue, hopelessness, constant worry, and lack of interest can be disruptive to the stability of a family. Understanding that depression may be an issue will help you and your partner better navigate and prepare for these problems.

When a partner or other family member is being treated for a mood disorder, you may not know the details of his emotional struggles or treatment.

It can be difficult for you when you feel left out of the loop on such an important matter that affects the whole family. You can try to get him to talk about issues that impact you and the family, using a respectful and gentle approach. Help him to realize that you are in this together. Try to understand that he may have times when he does not want to open up to you. But don't expect him to share the details of deeply private therapy conversations.

> You might feel lost and isolated yourself when a loved when has a mood disorder.

This is when a joint Family Meeting with his therapist may be beneficial to the health of your relationship and the entire family. A Family Meeting is simply a clinical appointment with his or her provider, such as his therapist, and the family member in treatment, you and perhaps other family members. It is done with your loved one's approval. A Family Meeting is meant to help everyone in the family understand the illness, how best to be supportive, answer questions, and clear the air of any underlying issues.

Effect on Children in the Family

A parent's or sibling's mental illness frequently affects the children in the family. This is true even if it's not spoken of openly in the home. Children usually observe the behavior and language of their parents and pick up on the subtle cues of depression. A child may also be at risk for developing depression later in life when raised in a family in which one parent has the illness. You might notice a change in your child's behavior, increased irritability, a change in schoolwork, or a different set of friends and interests.

Try to be open and honest with children in an age-appropriate way when a family member has a mood disorder. Children quickly pick up on the moods and behavior of a parent who is struggling with depression. Explain what's going on before their imaginations take over.

If you have a young child you might say, "Daddy's not feeling very well right now. He is very sad and has trouble doing some of the things he usually likes to do. We all have to be very patient now. He talked with his doctor and is getting medication so that he will feel better. He's going to be okay. He still loves you very much." The siblings of someone who has depression may need the same type of attention.

BURNOUT

Dealing with a mood disorder in a family member is a lot to handle. It requires patience, persistence, determination, and courage on your part. Try to be objective. Do your best to avoid getting caught up in the whirlwind of what your family member is saying and doing. Try to focus on her underlying feelings and emotional pain and respond to those. All of this can put pressure on you and other family members. It can lead to your own burnout unless you take steps to monitor and care for yourselves.

> Burnout is a state of emotional, physical, and mental exhaustion caused by prolonged stress.

What exactly is burnout? *Burnout* refers to the symptoms and emotions you may have from the stress of caring for someone. It's a kind of fatigue; the sense of having reached the limits of your endurance and your ability to cope. Burnout is the result of too many demands on your strength, resources, time, and energy. The situation goes beyond your ability to deal with it. Burnout is a fairly common experience among caregivers. When experiencing burnout, you may feel a combination of physical and emotional factors:

- Headaches
- Difficulty sleeping (insomnia)
- Lack of energy
- Muscle aches
- Stomach upsets
- Frustration, irritability, or anger
- Sadness
- Pessimism
- Resentfulness
- Disinterest and apathy
- Depression

How do you protect against burnout and keep from losing yourself in your family member's illness? The best way is to take time to care for yourself. Paying attention to your own needs does not mean you are ignoring your loved one's needs. Instead, it enables you to be a more available and productive support person.

Do your best to care for yourself physically, mentally, and emotionally. Try to get sufficient and regular sleep, exercise, and relaxation. Many caregivers find balance and relaxation in a yoga class or meditation exercises. Next, follow a balanced diet and nutrition plan as outlined in table 3.2. Keep a steady and consistent sleep schedule, and aim to get some physical exercise on most days of the week. Try to keep up with your own friends and support people, those who sustain you, and see them regularly—don't brush them aside for your caregiver role.

Pace yourself. Try to manage life's little daily stressors before they explode into unmanageable problems. You might break large tasks into smaller projects, prioritize the demands placed on you, and learn to say no on occasion. Saying "no" is hard for many of us, so you have to remind yourself that you cannot help your loved ones if you are stretched too thin.

Do your best to keep your usual routine and structure in your life. Make it a priority in your daily calendar. Look to your own needs and wants, doing what increases your own self-esteem and pleasure (hobbies, interests, skills, or volunteer work). These are what make your life rewarding and rich. Treat yourself to something special every once in a while—a meal out, a bouquet of flowers, a massage—and don't feel guilty doing so. Many people find it refreshing to take time for the Pleasurable Activities (see table 3.5).

Some people find brief supportive psychotherapy helpful at these times. This could be individual therapy or it might include joining a support group specifically for friends and families of those who have depression. You can find these groups within National Alliance on Mental Illness (NAMI) and Depression and Bipolar Support Alliance (DBSA), national organizations with local chapters that have small groups specifically for family members of those who have a mood disorder. There you will speak with others like yourself who find themselves in a similar situation with similar problems.

In this next story about Julia, I describe some of the ways that burnout can affect those of you who are in a caretaker role, which in turn can impact your ability to tend to the needs of your loved one. Taking steps to minimize the impact of full-time caregiving and pacing yourself are shown in this story.

Julia is a 53-year-old woman whose husband, Carlo, is receiving treatment for major depressive disorder. She has a full life with several hobbies, interests, and friends and works half time as a nurse. They have two grown children who live out of the house. Julia has become quite absorbed in the full-time care of her husband, who is now out of work. She takes it upon herself to gently remind him about taking his prescribed medications and keeping his therapy appointments, often driving him there herself. Julia tries, often unsuccessfully, to sit down and speak with Carlo about what's bothering him and feels frustrated when he doesn't respond to her or neglects his self-care routines. She is the chief cook and steward of their household, doing the laundry and errands, and attending to household repairs and bills, now that Carlo is so fatigued and no longer interested. Many of her prior activities and interests have been put on hold, including exercising and get-togethers with her friends, because of her all-consuming efforts to help her husband. She loves Carlo and wants to see him well and feels like she must not abandon him through this illness.

In the past month, Julia has felt fatigued, frustrated, and, at times, irritated with Carlo, which has put a strain on their marriage. Once or twice she has felt resentment for how his illness has affected her and their family. At times, Julia believes she has reached her limit and can no longer provide the care and support that he needs. She has experienced tension headaches, stomach upset, difficulty sleeping, and sore muscles, all of which is unusual for her.

Julia spoke with her family doctor, who recognized the signs of caretaker burnout and gave her some advice for coping with Carlo's illness in a healthier manner. He encouraged her to keep up with her own self-care routines, exercise, hobbies, and social events and to make caring for herself a priority. She was encouraged to restore relaxation and pleasurable activities back into her life, such as attending yoga class, getting her hair done, gardening, and having lunch with her friends, without feeling guilty. Her primary care physician also advised her to pace herself, to do only what she could realistically do and not try to do everything for everybody. This might include having to get other family members or friends engaged in helping Carlo to give her a break. It also includes learning how to say no to demands on her time and energy.

GUIDELINES IN CARING FOR YOURSELF

Rosen and Amador (1996) provide guidelines to help you care for yourself while in a support role:

- Learn all you can about the illness. The more you learn, the better you will be able to cope with it. A clear understanding may empower you to help your family member even more. Be an informed consumer: learn the facts, check the provider's credentials, and weigh the evidence on suggested treatment options.
- Have realistic expectations of how you can help. Set clear limits on what you can do, and try not to overcommit. Make sure your family member understands this.

- Give unconditional support to your family member who has depression.
- Aim for a regular routine in your own life. Work, eat, sleep, exercise, socialize, and relax. Keep those a priority and try not to allow your family member's needs to overshadow them.
- If you can, share your feelings about your life with your family member. Your ability to open up may go far in connecting with her.
- Don't take anything your family member says personally. Remember that she is seeing the world through a negative, distorted lens. Depression can impair her ability to express her thoughts, wishes, and needs. Try to understand that she may believe she is unlovable and unworthy of affection.
- Many caregivers find it useful to seek help from friends and other family members. This might include picking up the laundry, walking the dog, going to the post office, or taking the time to listen and support you. You cannot do this alone.
- Work together as a team with your family member. Avoid becoming a controlling force in her life.

Many people find success with the strategies learned in this chapter. Don't expect to master them all at once—pick one tactic at a time and work on that until you feel comfortable and then move on to another if you choose.

What if you have tried to do many of these things and find yourself feeling sad, down, or thinking that you, too, may be depressed? That is not common, but it can happen. Review the characteristic symptoms of depression discussed in chapter 1 to see how many of them apply to you and last two weeks or more. Then, try to follow the Basics of Mental Health outlined in chapter 3. This means you keep away from drugs and alcohol, keep a regular sleep pattern, eat a healthy diet, get daily physical exercise, aim for a routine and structure to your day, and avoid isolation. Aim for balance and a familiar routine in your life. Engage as much support for yourself as possible from your close friends and other family members. This may also be the time for you to speak with your primary care physician or family doctor, who will ask you questions about your emotional and physical health and assess your situation. You and she can then decide whether you need to see a mental health professional in the short term. Many people find a support group for family members like you to be particularly helpful as well.

18

Dos and Don'ts and Suggested Language

We each have our own way of coping with stressful situations and an illness like depression or bipolar disorder. Personal experiences from our past alters how we experience the illness, our relationships, our life events, and our work. As a result, we also have varying needs when it comes to receiving help from others. For some of us, receiving such help is a major challenge. It may make us feel vulnerable, needy, inadequate, or dependent. Others accept help much more easily. Try to remember this when you offer to help someone who has depression.

The table that follows offers some suggested language and approaches that many people have found useful. It may appear quite simple at first glance, but don't be fooled—a lot of key material is presented here. It can be a most useful reference or tool in your efforts to aid someone in distress. Some find it helpful to review each key point thoughtfully and slowly.

Instead of ...	Try to ...
Instead of offering advice ...	Listen. Be present and give your family member or friend your full attention.
Instead of judging your family member or friend ...	Listen. Say, "I wish it didn't have to be this way for you."
Instead of pressuring him to talk ...	Respect his choice about how much he wants to share. If someone confides in you, keep the conversation confidential.
Instead of blurting out reassuring words automatically when he expresses despair ...	Hold back. Think about whether you're only trying to calm your own anxiety.
Instead of abruptly saying, "Oh, you'll be fine" ...	Say, "I can see this is very difficult. I'm sorry." Validate his feelings as legitimate and make him feel heard and worthwhile.

Instead of . . .	Try to . . .
Instead of comparing his experience to your own or others . . .	Say, "I can see that you're in a lot of pain right now." Validate his feelings as legitimate and make him feel heard and worthwhile.
Instead of taking things too personally or resenting the time you are giving . . .	Provide unconditional love and support. Remember that greater patience and compassion may be necessary at times.
Instead of getting frustrated or setting low expectations for his recovery . . .	Maintain hope and a realistic optimism. Expect him to have good days and bad days, emotionally and physically.
Instead of promising him everything . . .	Only promise what you can deliver. Do what you say you are going to do.
Instead of silently blaming him for his illness, thoughts, or feelings . . .	Understand that this is a biologically based illness. Know the symptoms of depression and mania. Watch for the warning signs of worsening depression or mania and know when to encourage professional help.
Instead of being afraid to talk about depression or mania . . .	Respect your own limits. Educate yourself about the illness. Know the symptoms of depression and mania. Understand that talking about it can be helpful.
Instead of being afraid to ask him about suicidal thoughts, plans, or attempts . . .	Listen. Know that talking about it will not cause him to act. Be aware of the Warning Signs of Suicide. Call 9-1-1 if you are concerned.
Instead of taking over for him or treating him like a helpless person . . .	Offer to help in concrete, specific ways (picking up groceries, walking the dog, or going with him to an appointment). Look for ways to encourage his self-care.
Instead of avoiding him or making depression the focus of your relationship . . .	Include him in daily activities and social events. Let him be the one to determine if it's too much to manage. Keep your relationship as normal and balanced as possible.
Instead of trying to do everything for him . . .	Respect your own limits. Take care of yourself. You won't be effective at helping another person if you're burned out.

SUGGESTED LANGUAGE

Avoid Saying . . .

Despite your best intentions, the following phrases will *not* be motivating, and they will *not* have a positive effect on your loved one who has depression. They may make her feel less understood and invalidate her or make her feel that her troubles are not legitimate, not taken seriously, or dismissed by you. For these reasons, please try to avoid the following comments:

- It's not that bad.
- Things could be worse.
- Hang in there.
- There's light at the end of the tunnel.
- Things will get better.
- Just accept things the way they are.
- It's God's will.
- It's meant to be.
- It's time to get on with your life.
- Get over this and move on.
- You're not the only one who has problems.
- Buck up.

Instead, Try . . .

The following phrases will be more effective in offering your loved one comfort, support, and understanding. Please try to keep these in mind during your conversations:

- It sounds really bad. I'm sorry.
- I hear you.
- I can see that you're in a lot of pain right now.
- Tell me how I can help you.
- I'm with you. I'm here for you.
- This is really hard.
- For now, just hold on to one minute at a time.
- Just do what you can do for now.
- It's okay.
- This is going to take time.
- I wish it didn't have to be this way for you.
- I love you.

Conclusion

Thank you for taking this journey with me, for exploring ways you can help your loved one who has a mood disorder. In the process, I trust that you've improved your understanding of mood disorders and learned some new and effective skills. I hope that now having a better sense of what to say and do for your family member or friend who has depression or bipolar disorder will strengthen your efforts to aid in his recovery. Please know how much those of us who are affected by these illnesses appreciate your efforts.

The complex nature of your loved one's illness puts you in a difficult position as you struggle to find ways to help. The picture of a person's mood disorder can change over time as his episodes come and go, and you may find yourself having to interpret or "read" where he is along the course of his illness and respond accordingly. Caring for someone who has a mood disorder carries special challenges that make it different from caring for someone who has a physical medical problem (see chapter 6). Among these, for example, your loved one may have a lack of insight or unrealistic expectations surrounding his illness. He may reject your efforts to help or refuse to share confidential or detailed information about his situation from his providers. He may fear the stigma of mental illness and experience the painful loss of friends, self-esteem, or opportunities. All of this is on top of your need to remain emotionally neutral amid your loved one's angst and turmoil and somehow still be supportive and effective. You have a lot to juggle.

We started this journey by reviewing the basics of major depression and bipolar disorder and defining the common symptoms your loved one might experience. Most caregivers find this background information helps them better understand what they're dealing with and, in turn, how best to respond. We discussed how anxiety symptoms affect half of those who have depression. And you now have a sense of what to look out for if you suspect your family member or friend has a mood disorder. You'll be alert for changes from his usual self in general appearance, actions, thoughts, and feelings.

You now also have a better idea of how depression may differ in adults, adolescents, seniors, men, and women. Sometimes parents find it difficult to tell the difference between a normal teen stage your child is going through and actual depression—there is some crossover in symptoms. In your senior parents, grief or other medical conditions can often be confused with depression. Now you are more aware of what to look out for and when to call for professional help.

We then covered lifestyle interventions, the basic everyday things we all need to do that keep us both physically and emotionally healthy and are particularly important for your loved one who has a mood disorder. Paying attention to a healthy diet, regular sleep, exercise, daily routine and structure, and keeping up with other (supportive) people are all essential. You as a family member can be a role model by doing some or all of these things yourself and might be surprised that you feel more energized.

Following that, we discussed when to call for professional help, the different types of mental health providers and treatments available, and the importance of shared decision making. Options for paying for mental health treatment, with a brief overview of health insurance basics in the United States and what to do if your loved one cannot afford treatment, were presented. This has become an important and critical issue in recent times.

Along the way, I gave you some strategies to use every day. These are related to communication and support skills for interacting with your family member or friend and include nonjudgmental support, active listening, using open body language, asking open-ended questions, dealing with the negative thoughts, setting boundaries, or using tough love in your teen. One of the most effective skills to practice is the *empathic response*, a way to recognize and understand the emotions she's feeling and where they come from, putting yourself in the other person's shoes.

I shared with you the concept of *recovery*—the ongoing process of regaining control over one's life and all of its losses after receiving a psychiatric diagnosis—and described several definitions of recovery and what it looks like in a person. I also reviewed *well-being*, not only as an absence of illness or disease but also as a positive psychological function for health. That transitions to *resilience*, which is a person's ability to bounce back after a difficult time. When you foster resilience in your friend or family member who has depression, she is more likely to hardily weather the storms of depression and bipolar disorder. You as a role model can encourage her and teach her resilience skills.

Finally, I stressed the importance of taking care of yourself. Caring for a family member or a close friend who has any medical problem, particularly a mood disorder, is both stressful, time consuming, and fraught with worry. You can't help her if your energy and resources are spent or if you resent her illness. Take the time to get enough sleep, eat a balanced diet, get regular exercise, manage your stress, keep up with your own social contacts and activities, and pursue the hobbies that sustain you. Make sure you have some pleasurable experiences yourself each day and *pace yourself*. This may help you avoid burnout. Your family member or friend will thank you for this.

This book contains a lot of material. Don't expect to master it right away or after one reading. It takes time, practice, and patience to work on any new skill. I recommend you choose one or two approaches you think may be effective and work on each one slowly. Focus on one section of a chapter at a time. Read it as many times as needed. Once you feel comfortable using a skill, you may want to go on and learn a new one. You and the person you're helping will likely notice the difference—and feel better for it.

Good luck!

APPENDIX A

Medications

Here are some medications that can be used alone or in combination for depression, bipolar disorder, anxiety, and sleep (brand name is in parentheses).

Selective Serotonin Reuptake Inhibitors, or SSRIs
citalopram (Celexa)
escitalopram (Lexapro)
fluoxetine (Prozac)
fluvoxamine (Luvox)
paroxetine (Paxil)
sertraline (Zoloft)

Serotonin-Norepinephrine Reuptake Inhibitors, or SNRIs
desvenlafaxine (Pristiq)
duloxetine (Cymbalta)
venlafaxine (Effexor)

Other Antidepressants
bupropion (Wellbutrin)
mirtazapine (Remeron)

Tricyclic Antidepressants
amitriptyline (Elavil)
clomipramine (Anafranil)
imipramine (Tofranil)
nortriptyline (Pamelor)

Monoamine Oxidase Inhibitors, or MAOIs
phenelzine (Nardil)
tranylcypromine (Parnate)

Mood Stabilizers for Bipolar Disorder
carbamazepine (Tegretol)
lamotrigine (Lamictal)
lithium carbonate (Eskalith)
valproate (Depakote)

Atypical Antipsychotics
aripiprazole (Abilify)
brexpiprazole (Rexulti)
clozapine (Clozaril)
lurasidone (Latuda)
olanzapine (Zyprexa)
quetiapine (Seroquel)
risperidone (Risperdal)
ziprasidone (Geodon)

Antianxiety
alprazolam (Xanax)
buspirone (Buspar)
clonazepam (Klonopin)
lorazepam (Ativan)

Alternative Treatments, Nonprescription, Over the Counter
Folic acid
N-acetyl cysteine
Omega-3 fatty acids
S-adenosyl-L-methionine (SAMe)

Medications used for sleep
eszopiclone (Lunesta)
melatonin
ramelteon (Rozerem)
temazepam (Restoril)
trazodone (Desyrel)
zaleplon (Sonata)
zolpidem (Ambien)

Psychiatric Advance Directive

A Psychiatric Advance Directive (PAD) should include the following elements.

1. When it should be activated, under what conditions, with a description of the symptoms that makes a person unable to make decisions for himself.

2. The name and contact information of the person who will have decision-making authority and an alternate.

3. The person's preferred hospital if admission is necessary, with contact information. Also, hospitals and facilities where he or she would *not* want to go.

4. Who would and would not be allowed to visit the person at the facility or hospital.

5. Which treatments and medication is the person willing to receive and which is he or she not willing to try. Is the person willing to receive ECT (electroconvulsive therapy)?

6. List of effective ways of interacting with the person that are helpful; things that people can do.

Keep a separate Information Page with current contact information.

• Contact information for psychiatrist, therapist, PCP (primary care physician)

• Updated list of medications (including over the counter), allergies, dietary guidelines and restrictions, and other medical conditions

• Names and phone numbers of people the person wants to be contacted

• Information about his or her children, their schools, and routines

• Names of pets and how they should be taken care of

• Other useful information

Glossary

active listening A way to communicate that signals to a person that you are fully present and paying attention to what he is saying.

Affordable Care Act (ACA) A United States federal law passed in 2010 designed to make health insurance available to more people. Also known as Obamacare.

anxiety A feeling of excessive nervousness, apprehension, and worry about the future; the depth of worry, length of time it lasts, and how often it occurs that is out of proportion to the actual event.

automatic negative thoughts Thoughts that occur quickly and involuntarily during episodes of depression and cause distress. They arise because (1) negative events dominate the thinking of someone who has depression, and (2) the depressed mind tends to interpret and twist things in a negative direction. These thoughts don't accurately reflect reality.

behavioral activation A CBT skill and coping strategy for depression that can positively impact mood, decrease the risk for depression, and help to treat it. The aim of behavioral activation is to help a person re-engage in enjoyable, rewarding activities and develop or enhance his problem-solving skills.

bipolar depression A biologically based illness that negatively affects one's thoughts, emotions, and behaviors. It is relapsing and remitting yet treatable and alternates with episodes of extreme elevated mood (mania or hypomania). It affects relationships, activities, interests, and many other aspects of life. Bipolar depression is thought to involve a dysfunction of the network of *neurons* (brain cells) in the brain.

bipolar disorder A chronic mood disorder that has a major impact on daily life. Also known as *manic-depressive disorder*, it is thought to result from a dysfunction of the network of neurons in the brain. Bipolar disorder is characterized by episodes of extreme elevated mood or irritability (mania or hypomania) followed by episodes of depression.

boundaries Rules or limits on behavior that are agreed upon by you and the person who has depression.

bullying Unwanted and aggressive behavior toward another that involves a real or a perceived power imbalance, common in school-aged children and teens. Bullying includes making threats, spreading rumors and false information, attacking someone physically or verbally, and excluding someone from a group on purpose. It is often repeated over time. When bullying occurs over the internet and social media, it is known as cyberbullying.

Cognitive Behavioral Therapy (CBT) A kind of talk therapy, or *psychotherapy*, that addresses the connection between our thoughts, feelings, and actions. CBT teaches a person to identify and change thinking patterns that may be distorted, beliefs that are inaccurate, and behaviors that are unhelpful.

cognitive distortions Errors in thinking that twist a person's interpretation of an event. This is common in depression. CBT uses exercises to challenge and replace the negative and distorted thoughts with more realistic thoughts.

coping strategies The things we do to ease the stressors and challenges of daily life. Coping includes problem solving, self-soothing, relaxation, distraction, humor, mindfulness meditation, and other techniques.

delusions These are fixed false beliefs that can occur in some psychiatric illness.

depression A biologically based illness that negatively affects one's thoughts, emotions, and behaviors. Depression is a relapsing and remitting yet treatable illness of the mind and body. It affects relationships, activities, interests, and many other aspects of life. Depression is thought to involve a dysfunction of the network of neurons in the brain. This may happen when certain life experiences occur in a susceptible person. Also called unipolar or major depression.

difficult-to-treat depression Depression that continues to cause significant burden despite usual treatment efforts. It is a shift away from a goal of remission to optional symptom control and functional improvement.

distorted thinking Errors in thinking that twist someone's interpretation of an event. CBT uses a series of exercises to challenge and replace the negative and distorted thoughts that accompany depression.

dual diagnosis A term for those who experience a mental illness (like depression) and a substance use disorder at the same time.

empathic response A response that tries to identify with and understand someone's feelings or problems as if they were our own. We respond in a way that shows we recognize and understand what she is feeling and where it came from.

gene × environment A theory of depression that involves the interaction of our genes and the events in our life (our environment) that shape the complex network of cells in our brain.

hypomania An elevated, hyper mood that is part of bipolar disorder. It comes in episodes that alternate with bipolar depression, and the pattern is unique to each person. The symptoms are similar to mania. Hypomania is of shorter duration and less intense than mania.

major depression A treatable, biologically based illness that negatively affects one's thoughts, feelings, and behaviors. Depression is a relapsing and remitting illness of the mind and body. It affects relationships, activities, interests, and various other aspects of life. Depression is thought to involve a dysfunction of the network of neurons in the brain. This may happen when certain life experiences occur in a susceptible person.

mania An elevated, hyper mood that is part of bipolar disorder. It comes in episodes unique to each person and alternates with bipolar depression. The symptoms of elevated mood affect our thoughts, feelings, and behaviors. They include an inflated sense of self, increased physical energy, a decreased need for sleep, racing thoughts, irritability, high-risk behaviors, and others.

Mental Health First Aid A training program that teaches skills to help a person who has a mental health problem or is in a mental health crisis. It is given until appropriate professional treatment is received or the crisis resolves.

metabolic syndrome A physical condition that consists of having three of the following five cardiovascular risk factors: (1) central (around the midsection) obesity, (2) high blood pressure, (3) high levels of triglycerides (fat) in the blood, (4) low levels of the "good" HDL cholesterol, or (5) high levels of fasting blood sugar. Having metabolic syndrome puts you at increased chance of having a heart attack, stroke, or diabetes.

Mood Chart A way for a person to track fluctuations in her daily mood symptoms over time. It requires checking a box on a monthly form that best describes her mood for that day. It is a better reflection of the illness than relying on one's memory. When shared with her provider(s), they can use the information to decide on the best course of treatment.

mood disorders Conditions of the brain that involve the state of mind—the part of our inner self that colors and drives thoughts, feelings, and behaviors. Mood disorders are treatable biological illnesses. Mood disorders include major depression and bipolar disorder.

Obamacare A United States federal law passed in 2010 designed to make health insurance available to more people. Also known as the Affordable Care Act (ACA).

parity law A federal law in the United Stated that requires mental health and substance use disorders services coverage be comparable to medical/surgical coverage.

PCP Primary care physician, or the person's family doctor, internist or pediatrician.

postpartum depression Tearfulness, sadness, varying moods, irritability, and anxiety that peaks two to five days after childbirth and lasts about two weeks. It may be mild or deep and extreme and impairs functioning and the infant-caregiver attachment. Postpartum depression is related to a rapid shift in hormones following delivery that are experienced by the woman.

psychosis Indicates a severe illness and psychiatric emergency with periods of distorted thoughts and loss of touch with reality. The person may see or hear things that are not there, called hallucinations, which are very real to him. The concern is that he may act upon what he believes he is "told" to do. He may have paranoid delusions and believe that he is being stalked or followed.

realistic optimism A reasonable view of the future that involves hope and the confidence that, with enough hard work and determination, things will turn out well.

recovery A process of change through which individuals improve their health and wellness, live a self-directed life, and strive to reach their full potential. An ongoing process of gaining control of your life after a psychiatric diagnosis, and all of the losses that accompany it.

recurrence The return of full depressive symptoms following a *full recovery* from an episode of depression or bipolar disorder.

relapse The return of full depressive symptoms after *partial recovery* from an episode of depression or bipolar disorder.

remission Depressive symptoms completely cleared.

resilience The ability to face adversity and challenges (such as an illness like depression or bipolar disorder), adapt well, find solutions, and bounce back or recover more readily.

resilience factors A set of characteristics common to those who adapt well to stressful times.

response Partial improvement in symptoms and at least a 50 percent reduction in depression severity as measured by standardized rating questionnaires.

rumination When a person repeatedly thinks about the same thing.

shared decision making A process where your loved one and the clinician work together to make decisions and select diagnostic tests, treatments, and care plans based on clinical evidence while balancing the risks and benefits with his or her personal preferences and values.

sleep hygiene The personal habits, behaviors, and environmental conditions that affect a person's sleep. These include going to bed and waking up at the same time seven days a week, reserving the bed for sleep only, avoiding caffeine after noon, and more. These habits have a positive impact on the quality and quantity of sleep.

social media Websites and electronic applications that allow people to share photos, opinions, and events in real time and participate in electronic social networking. Some examples include FaceBook, Twitter, YouTube, Instagram, LinkedIn, as well as blogs and forums.

stigma An unfounded negative label or critical judgment placed on a person because of some characteristic, quality, or condition he has, such as mental illness; it may lead to being avoided, rejected, or shunned by others.

Suicide, Risk Factors for A set of personal life history items that may make it more likely that a person will take her life.

Suicide, Warning Signs A set of behaviors that may indicate a person is contemplating harming himself or taking his life.

support The time spent listening, hearing, and acknowledging the emotions that someone is experiencing. It also includes advocating on his behalf.

telehealth A general term for a broad array of technologies and tactics that deliver virtual medical visits (telemedicine) as well as other health services and health education.

telemedicine An online medical or mental health appointment in real time using applications on a computer or electronic device. It is similar to Skype or FaceTime where each person can see and hear the other. It is also called a virtual visit. It is not always paid for by private insurance companies or Medicare.

tough love A strategy of being firm yet loving, holding your loved one to agree on limits of behavior, and making him or her accountable for his wayward behavior and choices.

treatment-resistant depression Failure to respond or achieve remission after an adequate course of acceptable treatment of an adequate dose and duration of an antidepressant or other treatment (one or three or more courses of treatment—the number of treatment failures required to meet the definition of treatment resistance is not yet formally agreed upon).

triggers Events or circumstances that may cause someone distress and lead to an increase in symptoms of depression.

virtual visit An online medical or mental health appointment in real time using applications on a computer or electronic device. It is similar to Skype or FaceTime where each person can see and hear the other. It is also called telemedicine. It is not always paid for by private insurance companies or Medicare.

warning signs of depression Distinct changes from a person's usual thoughts, feelings, behaviors, routine, or self-care noticed by others. These changes may indicate a new or worsening episode of depression.

well-being Having a life that is meaningful, with purpose and direction, that is based on one's own beliefs and convictions, making use of personal talents and potential, where the person will manage life situations well, have positive relationships, and accept herself.

Resources

SOME OF THE MANY BOOKS
THAT MAY BE OF INTEREST

Herbert Benson. *The Relaxation Response*. Avon; 1975, revised 2000.

Norman T. Berlinger. *Rescuing Your Teenager from Depression*. HarperCollins; 2006.

David B. Burns. *Feeling Good: The New Mood Therapy*. HarperCollins; 2009.

Nell Casey. *Unholy Ghost: Writers on Depression*. William Morrow; 2001.

Adele Faber and Elaine Mazlish. *How to Talk So Teens Will Listen & Listen So Teens Will Talk*. William Morrow; 2005.

Roger Fisher and William Ury. *Getting to Yes: Negotiating Agreement without Giving In*. Penguin; 1983, 1991, 2012.

Felice Jacka. *Brain Changer: The Good Mental Health Diet*. Macmillan Australia; 2019.

Kay Redfield Jameson. *An Unquiet Mind: A Memoir of Mood and Madness*. Vintage Books; 1995.

Jon Kabat-Zinn. *Wherever You Go, There You Are: Mindfulness Meditation in Everyday Life*. Hyperion; 1994.

David J. Miklowitz. *The Bipolar Disorder Survival Guide: What You and Your Family Need to Know*. Guilford Press; 2010.

Francis Mark Mondimore. *Bipolar Disorder: A Guide for Patients and Families*. 3rd ed. Johns Hopkins University Press; 2014.

Francis Mark Mondimore. *Depression, the Mood Disease*. 3rd ed. Johns Hopkins University Press; 2006.

Francis Mark Mondimore and Patrick Kelly. *Adolescent Depression: A Guide for Parents*. 2nd edition. Johns Hopkins University Press; 2015.

Susan J. Noonan. *Managing Your Depression: What You Can Do to Feel Better*. Johns Hopkins University Press; 2013.

Susan J. Noonan. *Take Control of Your Depression: Strategies to Help You Feel Better Now*. Johns Hopkins University Press; 2018.

John J. Ratey with Eric Hagerman. *Spark: The Revolutionary New Science of Exercise and the Brain*. Little, Brown; 2008.

Laura Epstein Rosen and Xavier F. Amador. *When Someone You Love Is Depressed: How to Help Your Loved One without Losing Yourself*. Fireside; 1996.

Deborah Sichel and Jeanne Watson Driscoll. *Women's Moods: What Every Woman Must Know about Hormones, the Brain, and Emotional Health.* Quill; 1999.

Andrew Solomon. *The Noonday Demon: An Atlas of Depression.* Scribner; 2001.

Steven M. Southwick and Dennis S. Charney. *Resilience: The Science of Mastering Life's Greatest Challenges.* Cambridge University Press; 2012.

William Styron. *Darkness Visible: A Memoir of Madness.* Vintage Books; 1990.

William Ury. *Getting Past No: Negotiating in Difficult Situations.* Bantam; 1993, 2007.

Mark Williams, John Teasdale, Zindel Segal, and Jon Kabat-Zinn. *The Mindful Way through Depression: Freeing Yourself from Chronic Unhappiness.* Guilford Press; 2007.

ORGANIZATIONS THAT MAY BE OF INTEREST

American Foundation for Suicide Prevention (AFSP)
https://afsp.org
The AFSP funds research, provides educational programs for professionals, and educates the public about mood disorders and suicide prevention. It also promotes policies and legislation on suicide prevention and provides resources for survivors of suicide loss and people at risk.

Anxiety and Depression Association of America (ADAA)
https://adaa.org
The ADAA is an international organization dedicated to improving the lives of those who suffer from anxiety, obsessive-compulsive disorder, post-traumatic stress disorder, depression, and related disorders. It provides education, training, and research.

Beyond Blue
https://www.beyondblue.org.au
This website of the National Depression Initiative of Australia contains information for those with depression, anxiety, and suicide risk. Support comes in the form of telephone and online chat, email, and online forums.

Depression and Bipolar Support Alliance (DBSA)
https://dbsalliance.org
The DBSA's mission is to provide "hope, help, support, and education to improve the lives of people who have mood disorders." The DBSA has local

chapters with support groups that meet regularly, national educational
meetings, online wellness tools, an advocacy center, and training programs
for peer specialists. You can share ideas in its online community, the Facing
Us Clubhouse.

Depression and Bipolar Support Alliance (DBSA)
Balanced Mind Parent Network
https://www.dbsalliance.org/support/for-friends-family
/for-parents/balanced-mind-parent-network/
This network is a program of the DBSA. It serves to guide families raising
children with mood disorders to get the answers, support, and stability
they seek.

Families for Depression Awareness
www.familyaware.org
A national organization in the United States to help families recognize and
cope with depression and bipolar disorder, get people well, and prevent
suicides.

International Bipolar Foundation (IBPF)
https://ibpf.org
The goal of the IBPF is to improve the understanding and treatment of
bipolar disorder through research, to promote care and support resources
for individuals and caregivers, and to erase stigma through education.

Man Therapy
https://mantherapy.org
Using humor to show working-age men that talking about their problems
and getting help is not a sign of weakness, Man Therapy provides men, and
the people who care about them, information and resources about men's
mental health. They cover how to recognize signs and physical manifesta-
tions of stress, examine their own wellness, and connect with resources.

McMan's Depression and Bipolar Web
http://www.mcmanweb.com
This is a great website on depression and bipolar disorder run by John Mc-
Manamy, an award-winning journalist and author who has bipolar illness.

National Alliance for Mental Illness (NAMI)
https://www.nami.org
NAMI is the largest grassroots mental health organization in the United States. It provides information about mental illness, treatment options, support groups, and programs. You can go online to find a link to your local NAMI chapter. NAMI runs a highly regarded training program called Family to Family, a twelve-week evidence-based course on accepting and supporting those with mental illness. Approximately 300,000 people have completed it.

National Institute of Mental Health (NIMH)
www.nimh.nih.gov
This federal organization supports research on mental illness and provides information about depression and bipolar disorder, including current research and clinical trials.

Now Matters Now
https://www.nowmattersnow.org
This site offers tools for coping with suicidal thoughts; direct, easy-to-follow videos; and strategies to help those who have depression build more manageable and meaningful lives. As it was developed by Marsha Linehan, PhD, creator of Dialectical Behavior Therapy (DBT), it focuses on techniques such as mindfulness and paced breathing.

PsychEducation
https://psycheducation.org
This is an educational website run by Jim Phelps, MD, an active clinician and author with expertise in bipolar disorder and depression.

Suicide Prevention in College
https://www.affordablecollegesonline.org/college-resource-center/college-suicide-prevention/
This guide was designed to offer hope and help for those who are experiencing suicidal thoughts, as well as the friends and family who want so badly to help them.

Support for College Students with Bipolar Disorder
https://www.affordablecollegesonline.org/college-resource-center /college-student-bipolar-disorder/
This guide focuses on how students with bipolar disorder can find help on campus, the importance of continuing treatment plans, and how to make the college experience both a success and a wonderful time

This Is My Brave
https://thisismybrave.org
Its mission is to end the stigma of mental illness by sharing personal stories of people overcoming mental illness through poetry, essay, original music presented in live on-stage shows, stories published to its blog, and YouTube.

ONLINE INFORMATION THAT MAY BE OF INTEREST

American Psychological Association (APA)
The Road to Resilience
http://www.apa.org/helpcenter/road-resilience.aspx
This online brochure defines *resilience* as the "process of adapting well in the face of adversity, trauma, threats, and significant sources of stress— such as family and relationship problems, serious health problems, or workplace and financial stress." It provides personal strategies for developing and enhancing resilience.

Women's Mental Health
www.womensmentalhealth.org
This online library of articles, a blog, and newsletters sponsored by the Department of Psychiatry of the Massachusetts General Hospital (MGH) provides the latest information on mental health for women in all stages of life. The focus is primarily on mood disorders during the reproductive (childbearing) and menopausal years. There are also links to both the Clinical Program and the Research Program at the MGH Center for Women's Mental Health.

Physical Activity Guidelines
www.cdc.gov/physicalactivity
www.health.gov/PAGuidelines
These online sites contain guidelines on how much exercise you need at every age, how to add physical activity to your life, and how to measure the intensity of your physical exercise session.

United States Department of Agriculture (USDA)
Dietary Guidelines for Americans 2015–2020
www.health.gov/dietaryguidelines
www.choosemyplate.gov
These are the US sites for diet and nutritional guidance for all Americans. They include information on nutrients and their health benefits, portion sizes, weight management and calories, daily food plans, nutrition during pregnancy, physical activity, and interactive tools.

Mental Health First Aid (MHFA)
https://www.mentalhealthfirstaid.org
MHFA is a national program that teaches the skills to respond to the signs of mental illness and substance use. The 2016 guidelines for how to talk to someone who is suicidal can be found at https://mhfa.com.au/sites/default/files/MHFA_suicide_guidelinesA4%202014%20Revised.pdf.

References

Introduction

American Foundation for Suicide Prevention (AFSP). www.afsp.org/understanding -suicide/facts-and-figures. Accessed March 2019.

American Psychiatric Association (APA). *Diagnostic and Statistical Manual of Mental Disorders (DSM-5)*. 5th edition. American Psychiatric Association; 2013.

Lepine JP, Briley M. The increasing burden of depression. *Neuropsychiatr Dis Treat.* 2011;7(Suppl 1):3–7.

Martin LA, Neighbors HW, Griffith DM. The experience of symptoms of depression in men vs women: Analysis of the National Comorbidity Survey Replication. *JAMA Psychiatry.* 2013;70(10):1100–1106.

National Institute of Mental Health (NIMH). www.nimh.nih.gov. Accessed February 2019.

Mojtabal R, Olfson M, Han B. National trends in the prevalence and treatment of depression in adolescents and young adults. *Pediatrics.* 2016;138(6):12.

Wingo AP, Wrenn G, Pelletier T, Gutman AR, Bradley B, Ressler KJ. Moderating effects of resilience on depression in individuals with a history of childhood abuse or trauma exposure. *J Affect Disord.* 2010;126(30):411–414.

World Health Organization (WHO). www.who.int. Accessed February 2019.

Chapter 1. What Are Mood Disorders?

Altemus M. Neuroendocrine networks and functionality. *Psychiatr Clin North Am.* 2017;40(2):189–200.

American Psychiatric Association (APA). *Diagnostic and Statistical Manual of Mental Disorders (DSM-5)*. 5th edition. American Psychiatric Association; 2013.

Barker ED, Copeland W, Maughan B, Jaffee SR, Uher R. Relative impact of maternal depression and associated risk factors on offspring psychopathology. *Br J Psychiatry.* 2012;200(2):124–129.

Batten LA, Hernandez M, Pilowsky DJ, et al. Children of treatment-seeking mothers: A comparison with the sequenced treatment alternatives to relieve depression (STAR*D) child study. *J Am Acad Child Adolesc Psychiatry.* 2012;51(11):1185–1196.

Benbow A. Mental illness, stigma, and the media. *J Clin Psychiatry.* 2007;68(Suppl 2):31–35.

Bilello JA. Seeking an objective diagnosis of depression. *Biomark Med.* 2016;10(8):861–875.

Bromberger JT, Kravitz HM, Chang YF, Cyranowski JM, Brown C, Matthews KA. Major depression during and after the menopause transition: Study of Women's Health Across the Nation (SWAN). *Psychol Med.* 2011;41(9):1879–1888.

Bromberger JT, Schott L, Kravitz HM, Joffe H. Risk factors for major depression during midlife among a community sample of women with and without prior major depression: Are they the same or different? *Psychol Med.* 2015;45(8):1653–1664.

Cohen L, Freeman M. Psychiatric disorders in women: Diagnostic and treatment considerations across the female lifespan. An interactive CME course conducted by the Center for Women's Mental Health and the Psychiatry Academy, Department of Psychiatry, Massachusetts General Hospital; November–December 2019; Boston, MA.

di Scalea TL, Pearlstein T. Premenstrual dysphoric disorder. *Psychiatr Clin North Am.* 2017;40(2):201–216.

Fava GA, Rafanelli C, Grandi S, Conti S, Belluardo P. Prevention of recurrent depression with cognitive behavioral therapy: Preliminary findings. *Arch Gen Psychiatry.* 1998;55:816–820.

Frye MA. Bipolar disorder—a focus on depression. *N Engl J Med.* 2011;364(1):51–59.

Gambadauro P, Carli V, Hadlaczky G. Depressive symptoms among women with endometriosis: A systematic review and meta-analysis. *Am J Obstet Gynecol.* 2019; 220(3):230–241.

Hyde CL, Nagle MW, Tian C, et al. Identification of 15 genetic loci associated with risk of major depression in individuals of European descent. *Nat Genet.* 2016;48(9): 1031–1036. doi:10.1038/ng3623.

Johnson D, Dupuis G, Piche J, Clayborne Z, Colman I. Adult mental health outcomes of adolescent depression: A systematic review. *Depress Anxiety.* 2018;35(8):700–716.

Martin LA, Neighbors HW, Griffith DM. The experience of symptoms of depression in men vs women: Analysis of the National Comorbidity Survey Replication. *JAMA Psychiatry.* 2013;70(10):1100–1106.

Massachusetts General Hospital. MGH Center for Women's Mental Health. www.womensmentalhealth.org. Accessed February 2020.

McAllister-Williams RH, Arango C, Blier P, et al. The identification, assessment and management of difficult-to-treat depression: An international consensus statement. *J Affect Disord.* 2020;267:264–282.

Melton TH, Croarkin PE, Strawn JR, McClintock SM. Comorbid anxiety and depressive symptoms in children and adolescents: A systematic review and analysis. *J Psychiatr Pract.* 2016;22(2):84–98.

Nierenberg AA, DeCecco LM. Definitions of antidepressant treatment response, remission, nonresponse, partial response, and other relevant outcomes: A focus on treatment-resistant depression. *J Clin Psychiatry.* 2001;62(Suppl 16):5–9.

Nonacs R. NT-814: Neurokinin receptor antagonist effective for menopausal vasomotor symptoms. *MGH Center for Women's Mental Health*; March 12, 2020. https://womens mentalhealth.org/posts/nt-814-neurokinin-receptor-antagonist-effective-for -menopausal-vasomotor-symptoms/?utm_source=rss&utm_medium=rss&utm _campaign=nt-814-neurokinin-receptor-antagonist-effective-for-menopausal -vasomotor-symptoms. Accessed March 2020.

Park LT, Zarate CA Jr. Depression in the primary care setting. *N Engl J Med.* 2019;380(6): 559–568.

Pilowsky DJ, Wickramaratne, PJ, Rush AJ, et al. Children of currently depressed mothers: A STAR*D ancillary study. *J Clin Psychiatry.* 2006;67(1):126–136.

Regier DA, Rae DS, Narrow WE, Kaelber CT, Schatzberg AF. Prevalence of anxiety disorders and their comorbidity with mood and addictive disorders. *Br J Psychiatry Suppl.* 1998;(34):24–28.

Rice F, Riglin L, Lomax T, et al. Adolescent and adult differences in major depression symptom profiles. *J Affect Disord.* 2019;243:175–181.

Rush AJ, Aaronson ST, Demyttenaere K. *Aust N Z J Psych.* 2019;53(2):109–118.

Saveanu RV, Nemeroff CB. Etiology of depression: Genetic and environmental factors. *Psychiatr Clin North Am.* 2012;35:51–71.

Schmidt PJ, Ben Dor R, Martinez PE, et al. Effects of estradiol withdrawal on mood in women with past perimenopausal depression: A randomized clinical trial. *JAMA Psychiatry.* 2015;72(7):714–726.

Sichel D, Driscoll JW. *Women's Moods: What Every Woman Must Know about Hormones, the Brain, and Emotional Health.* Quill; 1999.

Soares C. Depression and menopause: An update on current knowledge and clinical management for this critical window. *Psychiatr Clin North Am.* 2017;40(2):239–254.

Stein MB, Sareen J. Generalized anxiety disorder. *N Engl J Med.* 2015;373(21):2059–2068.

Stewart DE, Vigod S. Postpartum depression. *N Engl J Med.* 2016;375(22):2177–2086.

Teasdale JD, Segal ZV, Williams JMG, Ridgeway VA, Soulsby JM, Lau MA. Prevention of relapse/recurrence in major depression by mindfulness-based cognitive therapy. *J Consul Clin Psychol.* 2000;8(4):615–623.

Trivedi MH, Rush AJ, Wisniewski SR, et al. Evaluation of outcomes with citalopram for depression using measurement-based care in STAR*D: Implication for clinical practice. *Am J Psychiatry.* 2006;163(1):28–40.

Trower M, Anderson RA, Ballantyne E, Joffe H, Kerr M, Pawsey S. Effects of NT-814, a dual neurokinin 1 and 3 receptor antagonist, on vasomotor symptoms in postmenopausal women: A placebo-controlled, randomized trial. *Menopause.* 2020;27(5).

Weissman MM, Feder A, Pilowsky DJ, et al. Depressed mothers coming to primary care: Maternal reports of problems with their children. *J Affect Disord.* 2004;78(2): 93–100.

Yeung A, Feldman G, Fava M. *Self-Management of Depression: A Manual for Mental Health and Primary Care Professionals.* Cambridge University Press; 2010.

Metabolic Syndrome

Akbaraly TN, Ancelin ML, Jaussent I, et al. Metabolic syndrome and onset of depressive symptoms in the elderly: Findings from the Three-City Study. *Diabetes Care.* 2011;34: 904–909.

Goldbacher EM, Bromberger J, Matthews KA. Lifetime history of major depression predicts the development of the metabolic syndrome in middle-aged women. *Psychosom Med.* 2009;71:266–272.

Kinder LS, Carnethon MR, Palaniappan LP, King AC, Fortmann SP. Depression and the metabolic syndrome in young adults: Findings from the Third National Health and Nutrition Examination Survey. *Psychosom Med.* 2004;66:316–322.

Marijnissen RM, Smits JE, Schoevers RA, et al. Association between metabolic syndrome and depressive symptom profiles—sex-specific? *J Affect Disord.* 2013;151(3):1138–1142.

Mendelson SD. *Metabolic Syndrome and Psychiatric Illness.* Elsevier; 2008.

Pan A, Keum N, Okereke OI, et al. Bidirectional association between depression and metabolic syndrome: A systematic review and meta-analysis of epidemiologic studies. *Diabetes Care.* 2012;35:1171–1180.

Rethorst CD, Bernstein I, Trivedi MH. Inflammation, obesity, and metabolic syndrome in depression: Analysis of the 2009–2010 National Health and Nutrition Examination Survey (NHANES). *J Clin Psychiatry.* 2014;75(12):e1428-1432.

Vaccarino V, McClure C, Johnson BD, et al. Depression, the metabolic syndrome and cardiovascular risk. *Psychosom Med.* 2008;70(1):40–80.

Chapter 2. Signs of Depression to Look For: Making the Diagnosis

Alpass FM, Neville S. Loneliness, health and depression in older males. *Aging Ment Health.* 2003;7(3):212–216.

Chapter 3. Healthy Ways to Handle Mood Disorders

Sleep

American Academy of Sleep Medicine. Healthy sleep habits. http://sleepeducation.org /essentials-in-sleep/healthy-sleep-habits. Accessed March 2019.

Asarnow LD, Manber R. Cognitive behavioral therapy for insomnia in depression. *Sleep Med Clin.* 2019;14(2):177–184.

National Institute of Neurologic Disorders and Stroke. Brain basics: Understanding sleep. NIH Publication No. 17-3440c. https://www.ninds.nih.gov/Disorders/Patient -Caregiver-Education/Understanding-Sleep. Accessed March 2019.

National Sleep Foundation. Sleep hygiene. https://www.sleepfoundation.org/articles /sleep-hygiene. Accessed March 2019.

Tsuno N, Besset S, Ritchie K. Sleep and depression. *J Clin Psychiatry.* 2005;66(10): 1254–1269.

Winkelman JW. How to identify and fix sleep problems: Better sleep, better mental health. *JAMA Psychiatry.* 2020;77(1):99–100. doi:10.100/jamapsychiatry.2019.3832.

Nutrition

Berk M, Jacka FN. Diet and depression—from confirmation to implementation. *JAMA.* 2019;321(9):842–843.

Bodnar LM, Wisner KL. Nutrition and depression: Implications for improving mental health among childbearing-aged women. *Biol Psychiatry.* 2005;58(9):679–685.

Diet and depression. *Tufts University Diet and Nutrition Letter.* Jan 2019;36(11):6–7.

Firth J, Marx W, Dash S, et al. The effects of dietary improvement on symptoms of depression and anxiety: A meta-analysis of randomized controlled trials. *Psychosom Med.* 2019;81(3):264–280. doi:10.1097/PSY.0000000000000673.

Frank E. Interpersonal and social rhythm therapy: A means of improving depression and preventing relapse in bipolar disorder. *J Clin Psychol.* 2007;63(5):463–473.

Jacka FN, O'Neil A, Opie R, et al. A randomized controlled trial of dietary improvement for adults with major depression (the "SMILES" trial). *BMC Med.* 2017;15(1):23. doi:10.1186/s12916-017-0791-y.

Jacka FN, Pasco JA, Mykletun A, et al. Association of Western and traditional diets with depression and anxiety in women. *Am J Psychiatry.* 2010;167(3):305–311.

Khalid S, Williams CM, Reynolds SA. Is there an association between diet and depression in children and adolescents? A systematic review. *Br J Nutr.* 2016;116(12): 2097–2108.

Ma J, Rosas LG, Lv N, et al. Effect of integrated behavioral weight loss treatment and problem-solving therapy on body mass index and depressive symptoms among patients with obesity and depression: The RAINBOW randomized clinical trial. *JAMA.* 2019;321(9):869–879. doi:10.1001/jama20190557.

Mayo Clinic. Mediterranean diet. www.mayoclinic.org/healthy-lifestyle/nutrition-and -healthy-eating/in-depth/mediterranean-diet/art-20047801. Accessed May 2019.

Sanchez-Villegas A, Delgado-Rodriguez M, Schlatter AA, et al. Association of the Mediterranean dietary pattern with the incidence of depression: The Seguimiento Universidad de Navarra/University of Navarro follow up. *Arch Gen Psychiatry.* 2009; 66(10):1090–1098.

United States Department of Agriculture (USDA). www.choose myplate.gov. Accessed March 2019.

United States Health and Human Services (HHS) and the United States Department of Agriculture (USDA). 2015–2020 Dietary guidelines for Americans. 8th edition. December 2015. http://health.gov/dietaryguidelines/2015/guidelines/. Accessed March 2019.

Physical Exercise

Carter T, Morres ID, Meade O, Callaghan P. The effect of exercise on depressive symptoms in adolescents: A systematic review and meta-analysis. *J Am Acad Child Adolesc Psychiatry*. 2016;55(7):580–590.

Choi KW, Chen CY, Stein MB, et al. Assessment of bidirectional relationships between physical activity and depression among adults: A 2-sample Mendelian randomization study. *JAMA Psychiatry*. 2019;76(4):399–408.

Cooney G, Dwan K, Mead G. Exercise for depression. *JAMA*. 2014;311(23):2432–2433.

Cooney GM, Dwan K, Greig CA, et al. Exercise for depression. *Cochrane Database Syst Rev*. 2013;9(9):CD004366.

Cotman CW, Berchtold NC, Christie LA. Exercise builds brain health: Key roles of growth factor cascades and inflammation. *Trends Neurosci*. 2007;30(9):464–472.

Dunn AL, Trivedi MH, Kampert JB, Clark CG, Chambliss HO. Exercise treatment for depression: Efficacy and dose response. *Am J Prev Med*. 2005;28(1):1–8.

Harvey SB, Øverland S, Hatch SL, Wessely S, Mykletun A, Hotopf M. Exercise and the prevention of depression: Results of the HUNT cohort study. *Am J Psychiatry*. 2018; 175(1):28–36.

Hoare E, Milton K, Foster C, Allender S. The associations between sedentary behaviour and mental health among adolescents: A systematic review. *Int J Behav Nutr Phys Act*. 2016;13(1):108.

Trivedi MH, Greer TL, Grannemann BD, et al. Exercise as an augmentation strategy for treatment of major depression. *J Psychiatr Pract*. 2006;12(4):205–213.

McMahon EM, Corcoran P, O'Regan G, et al. Physical activity in European adolescents and associations with anxiety, depression and well-being. *Eur Child Adolesc Psychiatry*. 2017;26(1):111–122.

Melo MCA, Daher EDF, Albuquerque SGC, de Bruin VMS. Exercise in bipolar patients: A systematic review. *J Affect Disord*. 2016;198:32–38.

Morres ID, Hatzigeorgiadis A, Stathi A, et al. Aerobic exercise for adult patients with major depressive disorder in mental health services: A systematic review and meta-analysis. *Depress Anxiety*. 2019;36(1):39–53.

Murri MB, Ekkekakis P, Menchetti M, et al. Physical exercise for late-life depression: Effects on symptom dimensions and time course. *J Affect Disord*. 2018;230:65–70.

Piercy KL, Troiano RP, Ballard RM, et al. The Physical Activity Guidelines for Americans. *JAMA*. 2018;320(19):2020–2028.

Rethorst CD, Trivedi MH. Evidence-based recommendations for the prescription of exercise for major depressive disorder. *J Psychiatr Pract*. 2013;19(3):204–212.

Rethorst CD, Wipfli BM, Landers DM. The antidepressant effect of exercise: A meta-analysis of randomized trials. *Sports Med*. 2009;39(6):491–511.

Schuch FB, Vancampfort D, Richards J, Rosenbaum S, Ward PB, Stubbs B. Exercise as a treatment for depression: A meta-analysis adjusting for publication bias. *J Psychiatr Res*. 2016;77:42–51.

United States Department of Health and Human Services (HHS). *Physical Activity Guidelines for Americans*. 2nd edition. HHS; 2018. https://health.gov/paguidelines/second -edition/pdf/Physical_Activity_Guidelines_2nd_edition.pdf. Accessed March 2019.

Vancampfort D, Stubbs B, Firth J, Van Damme T, Koyanagi A. Sedentary behavior and depressive symptoms among 67,077 adolescents aged 12–15 years from 30 low- and middle-income countries. *Int J Behav Nutr Phys Act.* 2018;15(1):73.

Yang L, Cao C, Kantor ED, et al. Trends in sedentary behavior among the US population, 2001–2016. *JAMA.* 2019;321(16):1587–1597.

Chapter 4. Finding Professional Help

Barry MJ, Edgman-Levitan S. Shared decision making—pinnacle of patient-centered care. *N Engl J Med.* 2012;366(9):780–781.

Elwyn G, Cochran N, Pignone, M. Shared decision making—the importance of diagnosing preferences. *JAMA Intern Med.* 2017;177(9):1239–1240.

Elwyn G, Frosch D, Thomson R, et al. Shared decision making: A model for clinical practice. *J Gen Intern Med.* 2012;27(10):1361–1367.doi.1007/s11606-012-2077-6.

Haselden M, Brister T, Robinson S, Covell N, Pauselli L, Dixon L. Effectiveness of the NAMI Homefront program for military and veteran families: In-person and online benefits. *Psychiatr Serv.* 2019;70(10):935–939. https://doi.org/10.1176/appi.ps.201800573.

Highet N, Thompson M, McNair B. Identifying depression in a family member: The carers' experience. *J Affect Disord.* 2005;87:25–33.

Mulley AG, Trimble C, Elwyn, G. Stop the silent misdiagnosis: Patients' preferences matter. *BMJ.* 2012;345:e6572.

Nierenberg AA. Medication Treatment of Bipolar Disorder: Challenges and Promises. Presented at: Patient and Family Education Day, The Dauten Family Center for Bipolar Treatment Innovation, Department of Psychiatry, Massachusetts General Hospital; June 23, 2018; Boston, MA.

Noonan SJ. *Managing Your Depression: What You Can Do to Feel Better.* Johns Hopkins University Press; 2013.

Psychiatric Advance Directives. National Resource Center on Psychiatric Advance Directives. https://www.nrc-pad.org. Accessed March 2019.

Sajatovic M, Jenkins JH, Cassidy KA, et al. Medication treatment perceptions, concerns and expectations among depressed individuals with type I bipolar disorder. *J Affect Disord.* 2009;115(3):360–366.

Simmons MB, Hetrick SE, Jorm AF. Making decisions about treatment for young people diagnosed with depressive disorders: A qualitative study of clinicians' experiences. *BMC Psychiatry.* 2013;13:335. doi:10.1186/1471-244X-13-335.

Sturmey, P. Behavioral activation is an evidence-based treatment for depression. *Behavior Modification.* 2009;33(6):818–829.

Swanson KA, Bastani R, Rubenstein LV, Meridith LS, Ford DE. Effect of mental health care and shared decision making on patient satisfaction in a community sample of patients with depression. *Med Care Res Rev.* 2007;64(4):416–430.

Weinstein S. Does your family know your mental health care preferences? Care for Your Mind. December 5, 2018. http://careforyourmind.org/does-your-family-know -your-mental-health-care-preferences. Accessed March 2019.

Chapter 5. Paying for Mental Health Treatment

Blumenthal D, Collins SR, Fowler EJ. The Affordable Care Act at 10 years–its coverage and access provisions. *N Engl J Med.* 2020;382(10):963–969.

Eibner C, Hussey PS. The Affordable Care Act in depth. RAND Health Care. https://www.rand.org/health-care/key-topics/health-policy/aca/in-depth.html. Accessed April 2019.

Frank RG. The creation of Medicare and Medicaid: The emergence of insurance and markets for mental health services. *Psychiatr Serv.* 2000;51(4):465–468.

Mark TL. The effect of the Affordable Care Act on uninsured rates among individuals with mental and substance use disorders. *Psychiatr Serv.* 2019;70(4):343.

Chapter 7. Support and Communication Strategies

Buckman R. *How to Break Bad News: A Guide for Health Care Professionals.* Johns Hopkins University Press; 1992.

Chapter 8. Helpful Approaches

Beck A, Rush A, Shaw BF, Emery G. *Cognitive Therapy of Depression.* Guilford Press; 1979.

Burns D. *Feeling Good: The New Mood Therapy.* HarperCollins; 2009.

Families for Depression Awareness. *Helping Someone Living with Depression or Bipolar Disorder: A Handbook for Families and Caregivers.* familyaware.org/new-caregiver-resources. Accessed March 2019.

Kitchener BA, Jorm AF. Mental health first aid training for the public: Evaluation of effects on knowledge, attitudes and helping behavior. *BMR Psychiatry.* 2002;2:10.

Langlands RL, Jorm AF, Kelly CM, Kitchener BA. First aid for depression: A Delphi consensus study with consumers, carers and clinicians. *J Affect Disord.* 2008;105:157–165.

Mental Health First Aid Australia. www.mhfa.com.au. Accessed May 2019.

Noonan SJ. *Managing Your Depression: What You Can Do to Feel Better.* Johns Hopkins University Press; 2013.

Noonan SJ. *Take Control of Your Depression: Strategies to Help You Feel Better Now.* Johns Hopkins University Press; 2018.

Reivich K, Shatte A. *The Resilience Factor.* Broadway Books; 2002.

Sheffield A. *How You Can Survive When They're Depressed.* Three Rivers Press; 1998.

Southwick SM, Charney DS. *Resilience: The Science of Mastering Life's Greatest Challenges.* Cambridge University Press; 2012.

Yeung A, Feldman G, Fava M. *Self-Management of Depression: A Manual for Mental Health and Primary Care Professionals.* Cambridge University Press; 2010.

Chapter 9. What You Can Do Now

Baldwin DS, Papakostas GI. Symptoms of fatigue and sleepiness in major depressive disorder. *J Clin Psychiatry.* 2006;67(Suppl 6):9–15.

Benson H. *The Relaxation Response.* 2000 revised edition. Avon; 1975.

Burns D. *Feeling Good: The New Mood Therapy.* HarperCollins; 2009.

Kabat-Zinn J. *Wherever You Go, There You Are.* Hyperion; 1994.

Noonan SJ. *Managing Your Depression: What You Can Do to Feel Better.* Johns Hopkins University Press; 2013.

Chapter 10. When Someone Is Suicidal

American Foundation for Suicide Prevention (AFSP). www.afsp.org/preventing-suicide/suicide-warning-signs. Accessed March 2019.

Beyer JL, Weisler RH. Suicide behaviors in bipolar disorder: A review and update for the clinician. *Psychiatr Clin North Am.* 2016;39(1):111–123.

Centers for Disease Control and Prevention (CDC). Suicide: Risk and protective factors. www.cdc.gov/violenceprevention/suicide/riskprotectivefactors. Accessed March 2019.

Centers for Disease Control and Prevention (CDC). www.cdc.gov. Accessed March 2019.

Centers for Disease Control and Prevention (CDC). *The relationship between bullying and suicide: What we know and what it means for schools.* 2014. https://www.cdc.gov /violenceprevention/pdf/bullying-suicide-translation-final-a.pdf. Accessed March 2020.

Centers for Disease Control and Prevention (CDC). *Youth Suicide Prevention Programs: A Resource Guide.* CDC; 1992.

Dazzi T, Gribble R, Wessely S, et al. Does asking about suicide and related behaviours induce suicidal ideation? What is the evidence? *Psychol Med.* 2014;44(16):3361–3363.

Fazel S, Runeson B. Suicide. *N Engl J Med.* 2020;382:266–274.

Harkavy-Friedman J. Ask Dr. Jill: Does mental illness play a role on suicide? American Foundation for Suicide Prevention. https://afsp.org/story/ask-dr-jill-does-mental -illness-play-a-role-in-suicide. Accessed May 2020.

Lardier DT Jr, Barrios VR, Garcia-Reid P, Reid RJ. Suicidal ideation among suburban adolescents: The influence of school bullying and other mediating risk factors. *J Child Adolesc Ment Health.* 2016;28(3):213–231.

McClatchey K, Murray J, Rowat A, Chouliara Z. Risk factors for suicide and suicidal behavior relevant to emergency health care settings: A systematic review of post-2007 reviews. *Suicide Life Threat Behav.* 2017;47(6):729–745.

Miron O, Yu K, Wilf-Miron R, Kohane IS. Suicide rates among adolescents and young adults in the United States, 2000–2017. *JAMA.* 2019;321(23):2362–2364.

Olson R. Why do people kill themselves? Centre for Suicide Prevention. 2014. https:// www.suicideinfo.ca/resource/suicidetheories/ Accessed April 2019.

Steinhauer JVA. Officials, and the nation, battle and unrelenting tide of veteran suicides. *New York Times.* April 14, 2019.

Stone DM, Simon TR, Fowler, KA, et al. Vital signs: Trends in state suicide rates—United States, 1999–2016 and circumstances contributing to suicide—27 states, 2015. *MMWR Morb Mortal Wkly Rep.* 2018;67(22):617–224. https://www.cdc.gov/mmwr /volumes/67/wr/pdfs/mm6722a1-H.pdf.

Turecki G, Brent DA. Suicide and suicidal behaviour. *Lancet.* 2016;387(10024):1227–1239.

National Institute of Mental Health (NIMH). www.nimh.nih.gov. Accessed March 2019.

National Suicide Prevention Lifeline. Suicide risk factors. www.suicidepreventionlife line.org. Accessed March 2019.

Youth Risk Behavior Survey 2017. Centers for Disease Control and Prevention. https:// www.cdc.gov/nchhstp/dear_colleague/2018/dcl-061418-YRBS.html. Accessed March 2019.

Chapter 11. Mood Disorders and Addictions

Blanco C, Alegria AA, Liu SM, et al. Differences among major depressive disorder with and without co-occurring substance use disorders and substance-induced depressive disorder: results from the National Epidemiologic Survey on Alcohol and Related Conditions. *J Clin Psychiatry.* 2012;73(6):865–873.

Di Forti M, Quattrone D, Freeman TP, et al. The contribution of cannabis use to variation in the incidence of psychotic disorder across Europe (EU-GEI): A multicentre case-control study. *Lancet Psychiatry.* 2019;6(5):427–436. doi:10.1016/S2215-0366(19)30048-3.

Gobbi G, Atkin T, Zytynski T, et al. Association of cannabis use in adolescence and risk of depression, anxiety, and suicidality in young adulthood: A systematic review and meta-analysis. *JAMA Psychiatry*. 2019:76(4);426–434.

Kessler RC. The epidemiology of dual diagnosis. *Biol Psychiatry*. 2004;56:730–737.

Mark TL. The costs of treating persons with depression and alcoholism compared with depression alone. *Psychiatr Serv*. 2003;54(8):1095–1097.

NAMI Chicago. Dual diagnosis: Mental illness and substance abuse. www.namichicago .org. Accessed April 2019.

NAMI. Dual diagnosis. https://www.nami.org/Learn-More/Mental-Health-Conditions /Related-Conditions/Dual-Diagnosis. Accessed April 2019.

SAMHSA. Behavioral health trends in the United States: Results from the 2014 National Survey on Drug Use and Health. https://www.samhsa.gov/data/sites/default/files /NSDUH-FRR1-2014/NSDUH-FRR1-2014.pdf Accessed April 2019.

Schrier LA, Harris SK, Kurland M, Knight JR. Substance use problems and associated psychiatric symptoms among adolescents in primary care. *Pediatrics*. 2003;111 (6 Pt 1):e699-705.

Chapter 12. For the Parents of a Teen or Young Adult and the Teens with an Affected Parent

Barry MJ, Edgman-Levitan, S. Shared decision making—pinnacle of patient-centered care. *N Engl J Med*. 2012;366(9):780–781.

Cheung AH, Zuckerbrot RA, Jensen PS, Laraque D, Stein REK; GLAD-PC Steering Group. Guidelines for adolescent depression in primary care (GLAD-PC): Part II. Treatment and ongoing management. *Pediatrics*. 2018:141(3).

Coles ME, Ravid A, Gibb B, George-Denn D, Bronstein LR, McLeod S. Adolescent mental health literacy: Young people's knowledge of depression and social anxiety disorder. *J Adolesc Health*. 2016;58(1):57–62.

Denizet-Lewis B. Why are more American teenagers than ever suffering from severe anxiety? *New York Times*. October 11, 2017. https://www.nytimes.com/2017/10/11 /magazine/why-are-more-american-teenagers-than-ever-suffering-from-severe -anxiety.html. Accessed March 2019.

Elwyn G, Cochran N, Pignone M. Shared decision making—the importance of diagnosing preferences. *JAMA Intern Med*. 2017;177(9):1239–1240.

Elwyn G, Frosch D, Thomson R, et al. Shared decision making: A model for clinical practice. *J Gen Intern Med*. 2012;27(10):1361–1367. doi:10.1007/s11606-012-2077-6.

Faber A, Mazlish, E. *How to Talk So Teens Will Listen & Listen So Teens Will Talk*. William Morrow; 2005.

Hoare E, Milton K, Foster C, Allender S. The association between sedentary behaviour and mental health among adolescents: A systematic review. *Int J Behav Nutr Phys Act*. 2016;13(1):108.

Johnco C, Rapee RM. Depression literacy and stigma influence how parents perceive and respond to adolescent depressive symptoms. *J Affect Disord*. 2018;241:599–607.

Khalid S, Williams CM, Reynolds SA. Is there an association between diet and depression in children and adolescents? A systematic review. *Br J Nutr*. 2016;116(12): 2097–2108.

Lardier DT Jr, Barrios VR, Garcia-Reid P, Reid RJ. Suicidal ideation among suburban adolescents: The influence of school bullying and other mediating risk factors. *J Child Adolesc Ment Health*. 2016;28(3):213–231.

Lipson SK, Lattie EG, Eisenberg D. Increased rates of mental health service utilization by U.S. college students: 10-year population-level trends (2007–2017). *Psychiatr Serv.* 2019;70:60–63.

Lovell S, Clifford M. Nonsuicidal self-injury of adolescents. *Clin Pediatr (Phila).* 2016;55(11): 1012–1019.

Marino C, Gini G, Vieno A, Spada MM. The associations between problematic Facebook use, psychological distress and well-being among adolescents and young adults: A systematic review and meta-analysis. *J Affect Disord.* 2018;225:274–281.

McMahon EM, Corcoran P, O'Regan G, et al. Physical activity in European adolescents and associations with anxiety, depression and well-being. *Eur Child Adolesc Psychiatry.* 2017;26(1):111–122.

Melton TH, Croarkin PE, Strawn JR, McClintock SM. Comorbid anxiety and depressive symptoms in children and adolescents: A systematic review and analysis. *J Psychiatr Pract.* 2016;22(2):84–98.

Schrier LA, Harris SK, Kurland M, Knight JR. Substance use problems and associated psychiatric symptoms among adolescents in primary care. *Pediatrics.* 2003;111 (6 Pt 1):e699-705.

Schrobsdorff, S. Teen depression and anxiety: Why the kids are not alright. *TIME.* October 27, 2016. http://time.com/4547322/american-teens-anxious-depressed -overwhelmed/. Accessed March 2019.

Simmons MB, Hetrick SE, Jorm AF. Making decisions about treatment for young people diagnosed with depressive disorders: A qualitative study of clinicians' experiences. *BMC Psychiatry.* 2013;13:335. doi:10.1186/1471-244X-13-335.

Swanson KA, Bastani R, Rubenstein LV, Meredith LS, Ford DE. Effect of mental health care and shared decision making on patient satisfaction in a community sample of patients with depression. *Med Care Res Rev.* 2007;64(4):416–430.

Vancampfort D, Stubbs B, Firth J, Van Damme T, Koyanagi A. Sedentary behavior and depressive symptoms among 67,077 adolescents aged 12–15 years from 30 low- and middle-income countries. *Int J Behav Nutr Phys Act.* 2018;15(1):73.

Wisdom JP, Clarke GN, Green CA. What teens want: Barriers to seeking care for depression. *Adm Policy Ment Health.* 2006;33(2):133–145.

Zuckerbrot RA, Cheung A, Jensen PS, Stein REK, Laraque D; GLAD-PC Steering Group. Guidelines for adolescent depression in primary care (GLAD-PC): Part I. Practice preparation, identification, assessment, and initial management. *Pediatrics.* 2018: 141(3).

Chapter 13. Technology in Mental Health

Bélanger RE, Akre C, Berchtold A, Michaud PA. A U-shaped association between intensity of internet use and adolescent health. *Pediatrics.* 2011;127(2)e330-335.

Best P, Manktelow R, Taylor B. Online communication, social media and adolescent wellbeing: A systemic narrative review. *Child Youth Serv Rev.* 2014:41:27–36.

BinDhim NF, Shaman AM, Trevena L, Basyouni MH, Pont LG, Alhawassi TM. Depression screening via a smartphone app: Cross-country user characteristics and feasibility. *J Am Med Inform Assoc.* 2015;22(1):29–34.

Cunningham JA, Gulliver A, Farrer L, Bennet K, Carron-Arthur B. Internet inter-ventions for mental health and addictions: Current findings and future directions. *Curr Psychiatry Rep.* 2014:16:521.

Grist R, Porter J, Stallard P. Mental health mobile apps for preadolescents and adolescents: A systematic review. *J Med Internet Res.* 2017;19(5):e176.

Horner S, Asher Y, Fireman GD. The impact and response to electronic bullying and traditional bullying among adolescents. *Comput Human Behav.* 2015:49:288–295.

Lardier DT Jr, Barrios VR, Garcia-Reid P, Reid RJ. Suicidal ideation among suburban adolescents: The influence of school bullying and other mediating risk factors. *J Child Adolesc Ment Health.* 2016;28(3):213–231.

Lenhart A. *Teens, Social Media and Technology Overview 2015.* Pew Internet and American Life Project; 2015.

Littlewood E, Duarte A, Hewitt G, et al. A randomised controlled trial of computerised cognitive behaviour therapy for the treatment of depression in primary care: The Randomised Evaluation of the Effectiveness and Acceptability of Computerised Therapy (REEACT) trial. *Health Technol Assess.* 2015;19(101):viii–171.

Marino C, Gini G, Vieno A, Spada MM. The associations between problematic Facebook use, psychological distress and well-being among adolescents and young adults: A systematic review and meta-analysis. *J Affect Disord.* 2018;225:274–281.

Miner AS, Milstein A, Schuller S, et al. Smartphone-based conversational agents and responses to questions about mental health, interpersonal violence and physical health. *JAMA Intern Med.* 2016:176(5):619–625.

O'Keefe GS, Clarke-Pearson K, and Council on Communications and Media. The impact of social media on children, adolescents, and families. *Pediatrics.* 2011;127(4):800–804.

Radovic A, Vona PL, Santostefano AM, Ciaravino S, Miller E, Stein BD. Smartphone applications for mental health. *Cyberpsychol Behav Soc Netw.* 2016;19(7):465–470.

Stasiak K, Fleming T, Lucassen ME, Shepherd MJ, Whittaker R, Merry SN. Computer-based and online therapy for depression and anxiety in children and adolescents. *J Child Adolesc Psychopharmacol.* 2016;26(3):235–245.

Chapter 14. Depression in a Seniors

Mojtabai R. Diagnosing depression in older adults in primary care. *N Engl J Med.* 2014; 370(13):1180–1182.

Qata D, Ozenbergweger K, Olfson M. Prevalence of prescriptions with depression as a potential adverse effect among adults in the United States. *JAMA.* 2018;319(22): 2289–2298.

Taylor WD. Depression in the elderly. *N Engl J Med.* 2014;371(13);11228–11236.

Chapter 15. What Recovery Looks Like

Anthony WA. Recovery from mental illness: The guiding vision of the mental health system in the 1990s. *Psychosoc Rehabil J.* 1993;16:11–23.

DBSA/Appalachian Consulting Group. *DBSA Peer Specialist Core Training Manual.* 2009;2:2.

Manderscheld RW, Ryff CD, Freeman EJ, McKnight-Eily LR, Dhingra S, Strine TW. Evolving definitions of mental illness and wellness. *Prev Chronic Dis.* 2010;7(1):1–6.

National Association of Mental Illness (NAMI). Can people recover from mental illness. https://www.nami.org/FAQ/General-Information-FAQ/Can-people-recover-from -mental-illness-Is-there-a. Accessed March 2019.

Ryff CD. Psychological well-being revisited: Advances in science and practice of eudaimonia. *Psychother Psychosom.* 2014;83(1):10–28. doi:10.1159/000353263.

SAMHSA Working Definition of Recovery. https://store.samhsa.gov/system/files/pep12 -recdef.pdf. Accessed March 2019.

Well Beyond Blue: Report of the externally-led patient-focused medical product development meeting on major depressive disorder. DBSA. March 2019. https://www.dbsalliance.org/wp-content/uploads/2019/10/final-Externally-led-VOPR.pdf Accessed January 2020.

Chapter 16. Anticipating Recovery: Skills to Have in Place

American Psychological Association (APA). Resilience guide for parents and teachers. www.apa.org/helpcenter/resilience.aspx. Accessed May 2015.

American Psychological Association (APA). The road to resilience. www.apa.org/helpcenter/road-resilience.aspx. Accessed March 2020.

Catalano D, Wilson L, Chan F, Chiu C, Muller VR. The buffering effect of resilience on depression among individuals with spinal cord injury: A structural equation model. *Rehabil Psychol.* 2011;56(3):200–211.

Comas-Diaz L, Luthar SS, Maddi SR, O'Neill HK, Saakvitne KW, Tedeschi RG. *The Road to Resilience.* American Psychological Association, 2013.

Dunn AL, Trivedi MH, Kampert JB, Clark CG, Chamblis HO. Exercise treatment for depression: Efficacy and dose response. *Am J Prev Med.* 2005;28(1):1–8.

Haeffel GF, Vargas I. Resilience to depressive symptoms: The buffering effects of enhancing cognitive style and positive life events. *J Behav Ther Exp Psychiatry.* 2011;42(1):13–18.

Mak WWS, Ng ISW, Wong CCY. Resilience: Enhancing well-being through the positive cognitive triad. *J Couns Psychol.* 2011;58(4):610–617.

Masten AS. Ordinary magic: Resilience processes in development. *Am Psychol.* 2001;56:227–238.

Mead GE, Morley W, Campbell P, Greig CA, McMurdo M, Lawlor DA. Exercise for depression. *Cochrane Database of Syst Rev.* 2009;(3):CD004366.

Rethorst CD, Trivedi MH. Evidence-based recommendations for the prescription of exercise for major depressive disorder. *J Psychiatr Pract.* 2013;19(3):204–212.

Southwick SM, Charney DS. *Resilience: The Science of Mastering Life's Greatest Challenges.* Cambridge University Press; 2012.

Stein MB, Campbell-Sills L, Gelernter J. Genetic variation in 5HTTLPR is associated with emotional resilience. *Am J Med Genet B Neuropsychiatr Genet.* 2009;150B(7):900–906.

Trivedi MH, Greer TL, Grannemann BD, Chambliss HO, Jordan AN. Exercise as an augmentation strategy for treatment of major depression. *J Psychiatr Pract.* 2006;12(4):205–213.

Vanderhorst RK, McLaren S. Social relationships as predictors of depression and suicidal ideation in older adults. *Aging Ment Health.* 2005;9(6):517–525.

Wingo AP, Wrenn G, Pelletier T, Gutman AR, Bradley B, Ressler KJ. Moderating effects of resilience on depression in individuals with a history of childhood abuse or trauma exposure. *J Affect Disord.* 2010;126(30):411–414.

Chapter 17. Caring for the Caregivers

Barker ED, Copeland W, Maughan B, Jaffee SR, Uher R. Relative impact of maternal depression and associated risk factors on offspring psychopathology. *Br J Psychiatry.* 2012;200(2):124–129.

Batten LA, Hernandez M, Pilowsky DJ, et al. Children of treatment-seeking mothers: A comparison with the sequenced treatment alternatives to relieve depression (STAR*D) child study. *J Am Acad Child Adolesc Psychiatry.* 2012;51(11):1185–1196.

DePaulo JR Jr, Horvitz LA. *Understanding Depression: What We Know and What You Can Do about It.* John Wiley and Sons; 2002.

Golant M, Golant S. *What to Do When Someone You Love Is Depressed.* Henry Holt; 1996, 2007.

Pilowsky DJ, Wickramaratne PJ, Rush AJ, et al. Children of currently depressed mothers: A STAR*D ancillary study. *J Clin Psychiatry.* 2006;67(1):126–136.

Rosen LE, Amador XF. *When Someone You Love Is Depressed: How to Help Your Loved One without Losing Yourself.* Simon & Shuster; 1996.

Weissman MM, Feder A, Pilowsky DJ, et al. Depressed mothers coming to primary care: Maternal reports of problems with their children. *J Affect Disord.* 2004;78(2):93–100.

Weissman MM, Wickramaratne P, Pilowsky DJ, et al. Treatment of maternal depression in a medication clinical trial and its effect on children. *Am J Psychiatry.* 2015;172(5): 450–459.

Chapter 18. Dos and Don'ts and Suggested Language

Yeung A, Feldman G, Fava M. *Self-Management of Depression: A Manual for Mental Health and Primary Care Professionals.* Cambridge University Press; 2010, appendix C.

Index

Page numbers in *italics* refer to tables.